CORTISOL DETOX PLAN
7 DAYS TO RESET, 14 DAYS TO TRANSFORM
A Natural Guide to Balance Hormones, Reduce Stress and Boost Energy

Liv Marwin

Copyright © 2025 Liv Marwin - All Rights Reserved

All rights reserved. No part of this book may be reproduced, distributed, transmitted, or stored in any form or by any means without the prior written permission of the author or publisher, except as permitted by applicable copyright law.

Under no circumstances shall the author or publisher be held liable for any damages, financial losses, or claims arising from the use of the information contained in this book, whether directly or indirectly.

Legal Notice:
This book is protected under copyright law and is intended solely for personal use. You may not copy, modify, sell, distribute, or reproduce any part of this book without explicit written consent from the author or publisher.

Disclaimer:
The information provided in this book is for educational and informational purposes only. While every effort has been made to ensure the content is accurate and up-to-date, no guarantees or warranties of any kind are expressed or implied. Readers acknowledge that the author is not providing professional legal, medical, financial, or other advice. The information in this book has been compiled from various sources, and readers are advised to consult a qualified professional before applying any techniques described.

By reading this book, you agree that the author shall not be held responsible for any direct or indirect losses, damages, or consequences resulting from the use of the content herein, including but not limited to errors, omissions, or inaccuracies.

TABLE OF CONTENTS

INTRODUCTION: RECLAIMING BALANCE IN A WORLD THAT NEVER PAUSES ... 7
- *Why Stress Isn't Just Mental—It's Hormonal* ... 7
- *The Shift Toward Intentional Living* ... 7
- *What It Means to Detox Your Stress Response* ... 7
- *A New Framework for Lasting Change* ... 7
- *Why Now Is the Time to Take Back Control* ... 8
- *Moving Forward—One Step at a Time* ... 8

CHAPTER 1: UNDERSTANDING CORTISOL ... 9
1.1 What is Cortisol and Why Is It Important? ... 9
- *The "Engine" of Your Body: Why Cortisol Is Crucial* ... 9
- *Cortisol as the "Stress Hormone"* ... 9
- *The Modern Lifestyle and Its Impact on Cortisol Balance* ... 9
- *The Role of Cortisol in Your Body's Functions* ... 10
- *How Chronic Stress Affects Your Health* ... 10

1.2 Signs and Causes of Cortisol Imbalance ... 11
- *Triggers of Cortisol Dysregulation: Poor Diet, Sleep Deprivation, Chronic Stress* ... 11
- *Symptoms of High Cortisol: Anxiety, Weight Gain, Insomnia, Fatigue* ... 11
- *Symptoms of Low Cortisol: Chronic Fatigue, Apathy, Lack of Energy* ... 12
- *The Importance of Recognizing Early Warning Signs* ... 12

1.3 How to Test and Monitor Cortisol Levels ... 12
- *Lab Tests: Saliva, Blood, and Urine – Which Works Best?* ... 13
- *At-Home Testing Kits: Accuracy and Convenience* ... 14
- *Understanding Your Results: When to Take Action* ... 14
- *Recognizing Patterns, Not Just Numbers* ... 14
- *When Testing Becomes Essential* ... 15

1.4 Why Do a Cortisol Detox? ... 15
- *The Negative Effects of Cortisol Overload* ... 15
- *The Benefits of a Detox: Reclaiming Balance* ... 16
- *How This Detox Can Transform Your Life* ... 17
- *A Holistic Approach to Healing* ... 17

CHAPTER 2: THE FOUNDATIONS OF CORTISOL DETOX ... 19
2.1 Preparing for Change ... 19
- *Measuring Your Stress Levels: A Simple Starting Point* ... 19
- *Essential Tools for Success: Journals, Planners, and Basic Ingredients* ... 20
- *Taking the Initial Test: Understanding Your Current State* ... 20
- *Building Your Foundation for Change* ... 21

2.2 The Nine Pillars of Cortisol Detox ... 21
- *1. Nutrition: Foods That Help Regulate Cortisol* ... 21
- *2. Lifestyle: Sleep, Movement, and Stress Management* ... 21
- *3. Natural Remedies: Adaptogens, Aromatherapy, and Supplements* ... 22
- *4. Hydration: The Importance of Functional Beverages* ... 22
- *5. Environmental Changes: Creating a Calm Living Space* ... 22
- *6. Circadian Rhythm: Aligning Your Body Clock with Nature* ... 23
- *7. Mindfulness Practices: Gratitude, Meditation, and Journaling* ... 23
- *8. Nature Connection: Reaping the Benefits of Outdoor Activities* ... 23
- *9. Play and Creativity: The Stress-Relief Power of Joy* ... 23

CHAPTER 3: THE DETOX NUTRITION PLAN ... 25
3.1 Foods That Help and Hurt Cortisol Levels ... 25
- *Cortisol-Friendly Foods: Nutrients That Nourish Balance* ... 25
- *Foods to Avoid: Cortisol Triggers in Your Diet* ... 26
- *How to Combine Foods for Steady Energy and Lower Stress* ... 26
- *Final Thoughts on Food as Medicine* ... 27

3.2 Recipes to Support Cortisol Balance ... 27
- *Breakfasts: stress-busting starts to your day* ... 27
- *Lunches: anti-inflammatory and satisfying meals* ... 33

Dinners: restorative and healing meals 40
Snacks: quick boosts for energy and calm 49
Smoothies for Stress Relief and Hormonal Balance 54
Quick and Easy Meal Prep Tips 61

CHAPTER 4: THE 7-DAY RESET PLAN 63
4.1 How to Start Your Detox Journey 63
Setting Up Your Daily Routine: Morning, Afternoon, and Evening Practices 63
Overcoming Common Challenges in the First Week 64
4.2 The 7-Day Plan 65
Day 1: Awakening Awareness 65
Day 2: Detox and Release 66
Day 3: Grounding and Stability 66
Day 4: Rejuvenation and Renewal 66
Day 5: Strength and Energy 67
Day 6: Clarity and Focus 67
Day 7: Reflection and Renewal 67

CHAPTER 5: THE 14-DAY TRANSFORMATION PLAN 69
5.1 Week One: Building the Foundation 69
Laying the Groundwork for Lasting Change 69
Solidifying New Habits for Nutrition 69
Movement: Building Strength and Flexibility 70
Prioritizing Restorative Sleep 70
Creating a Stress-Resilient Routine 70
Reinforcing Progress Through Reflection 71
Final Thoughts on Week One 71
5.2 Week Two: Advanced Strategies 71
Taking Growth to the Next Level 71
Emotional Well-Being: Strengthening Relationships and Reducing Mental Stress 71
Incorporating Creativity and Play into Your Routine 72
Adapting the Plan to Fit Your Lifestyle and Goals 73
Sustaining Growth Beyond the Two Weeks 73

CHAPTER 6: DAILY ROUTINES FOR CORTISOL BALANCE 75
6.1 Crafting Your Morning Routine 75
The Importance of a Grounded Morning 75
Step 1: Breathing Exercises to Start the Day 75
Step 2: Journaling for Mental Clarity 76
Step 3: Energizing Yet Stress-Free Breakfast Options 76
Step 4: Sunlight and Movement for Cortisol Regulation 76
Step 5: Morning Rituals to Limit Technology Stress 76
Step 6: Hydration for Hormonal Balance 77
Step 7: Setting Intentions and Affirmations 77
Closing Morning Routine Thoughts 77
6.2 Midday Strategies for Energy and Focus 77
Avoiding Blood Sugar Spikes and Midday Slumps 77
Quick Mindfulness Breaks to Reset Mental Focus 78
Stretching and Movement for Energy and Circulation 79
Hydration for Cortisol Regulation 79
Sustaining Energy Without Stimulants 79
6.3 Evening Relaxation Techniques 80
Unwinding with Aromatherapy and Warm Baths 80
Breathwork and Meditation for Nervous System Reset 80
Calming Activities That Promote Stillness 81
Pre-Bedtime Rituals for Better Sleep 81
Sound Therapy and Nature Sounds for Deeper Sleep 81
Creating a Consistent Sleep Schedule 82
Final Touchpoints for Evening Calm 82

6.4 Making Habits Stick for the Long Term 82
- *Tips for Building Consistent and Sustainable Routines* 82
- *How to Handle Setbacks* 83
- *Practical Tools for Long-Term Success* 84
- *Building a Resilient Mindset* 84
- *Final Thoughts on Long-Term Change* 84

CHAPTER 7: NATURAL SUPPORT FOR STRESS REDUCTION 85
7.1 Herbs and Adaptogens for Cortisol Balance 85
- *Ashwagandha: The Root of Calm Resilience* 85
- *Rhodiola Rosea: The Energy Restorer* 86
- *Ginseng: The Energy Booster* 86
- *Holy Basil: The Stress Reliever* 86
- *How to Use Herbs Safely and Effectively* 87

7.2 Supplements and Essential Oils 87
- *Magnesium: The Relaxation Mineral* 87
- *Omega-3 Fatty Acids: Brain and Mood Stabilizers* 88
- *Vitamin C: The Stress Shield* 88
- *Essential Oils: Aromatic Stress Relievers* 89
- *Combining Supplements and Essential Oils for Synergy* 89
- *Practical Tips for Daily Use* 89

7.3 DIY Remedies 89
- *Stress-Relief Scrubs: Exfoliation Meets Relaxation* 90
- *Bath Rituals: Immersive Relaxation Therapy* 91
- *Herbal Teas: Sipping Calmness* 91
- *Aromatherapy Blends: Portable Calm* 92
- *Personalizing Your DIY Remedies* 92

CHAPTER 8: LONG-TERM STRATEGIES FOR A LOW-STRESS LIFE 93
8.1 Designing an Anti-Stress Lifestyle 93
- *Recognizing and Avoiding Hidden Stress Triggers* 93
- *The Power of Scheduled Rest and Regenerative Breaks* 94
- *Creating a Holistic Stress-Management Framework* 94
- *The Role of Consistency in Stress Resilience* 95
- *Final Thoughts on Designing an Anti-Stress Lifestyle* 95

8.2 The Role of Healthy Relationships and Community 95
- *The Biological and Psychological Benefits of Healthy Relationships* 95
- *Building Positive Connections: The Art of Nurturing Relationships* 96
- *The Role of Community in Reducing Stress* 97
- *Navigating Toxic Relationships* 97

8.3 Celebrating Progress and Staying Motivated 98
- *Redefining Success: Beyond the Scale and Surface-Level Goals* 98
- *The Power of Small Wins: Building Momentum Through Tiny Victories* 99
- *Staying Motivated During Plateaus and Setbacks* 99
- *Building a Reward System That Fuels Progress* 100
- *Finding Inspiration Through Role Models and Accountability* 100

CONCLUSIONS 101
- *Maintaining Balance After the Detox* 101
- *Sustaining the Rituals That Anchor You* 101
- *Recognizing Stress Before It Escalates* 101
- *Adopting a Growth Mindset* 102
- *Investing in Personal Development* 102
- *Celebrating Milestones to Reinforce Growth* 102
- *Returning to Your Foundation* 102

Acknowledgements 103

INTRODUCTION: RECLAIMING BALANCE IN A WORLD THAT NEVER PAUSES

Modern life moves fast—too fast. Between endless notifications, packed schedules, and the pressure to DO MORE, it's no wonder that STRESS has become a constant companion for so many. Yet, despite its familiarity, stress is often misunderstood. It's not just a TEMPORARY INCONVENIENCE or a BADGE OF HONOR signaling ambition. It's a BIOLOGICAL RESPONSE with far-reaching effects on the BODY, MIND, and SPIRIT.

This book is an invitation to step off the treadmill of CONSTANT URGENCY and into a space where CALM isn't just an occasional break—it's A WAY OF LIFE.

WHY STRESS ISN'T JUST MENTAL—IT'S HORMONAL

Stress isn't all in your HEAD. It's deeply tied to your HORMONAL SYSTEM, especially CORTISOL—the body's PRIMARY STRESS HORMONE. While cortisol serves a CRITICAL PURPOSE in survival, helping you respond to danger, the problem begins when it DOESN'T SHUT OFF.

CHRONIC STRESS turns what's meant to be a SHORT-TERM DEFENSE MECHANISM into a LONG-TERM HEALTH THREAT. It can DISRUPT SLEEP, WEAKEN IMMUNITY, FUEL INFLAMMATION, and even lead to HORMONAL IMBALANCES that affect MOOD, WEIGHT, and ENERGY LEVELS.

But here's the good news—your BIOLOGY ISN'T FIXED. The body is DESIGNED TO HEAL, and with the right tools, you can RESET YOUR STRESS RESPONSE, REBALANCE YOUR HORMONES, and reclaim the CALM you deserve.

THE SHIFT TOWARD INTENTIONAL LIVING

Creating a LOW-STRESS LIFE isn't about ESCAPING REALITY. It's about learning to NAVIGATE REALITY with CLARITY, CONFIDENCE, and INTENTION. Stress isn't always avoidable, but how you RESPOND to it can change everything.

Imagine waking up feeling REFRESHED instead of DRAINED. Picture yourself moving through challenges with a sense of STEADINESS, even when things feel uncertain. These outcomes aren't reserved for the LUCKY FEW. They're ACHIEVABLE, and they start with INTENTIONAL CHOICES.

This book isn't about chasing QUICK FIXES or TEMPORARY RELIEF. It's about building a SUSTAINABLE FOUNDATION that supports LONG-TERM BALANCE.

WHAT IT MEANS TO DETOX YOUR STRESS RESPONSE

Detoxing isn't just about FOOD or TOXINS. It's about clearing out MENTAL CLUTTER, EMOTIONAL BAGGAGE, and PHYSICAL HABITS that keep you stuck in a STATE OF TENSION. Think of it as RESETTING YOUR INTERNAL COMPASS—realigning your habits, mindset, and daily rhythms to reflect your HIGHEST PRIORITIES.

This process is both PRACTICAL and PERSONAL. It's not a rigid formula but a FLEXIBLE FRAMEWORK that adapts to YOUR LIFESTYLE and NEEDS. Whether you're looking to REGAIN ENERGY, IMPROVE FOCUS, or simply BREATHE EASIER, this book provides tools to help you START WHERE YOU ARE and GROW INTENTIONALLY.

A NEW FRAMEWORK FOR LASTING CHANGE

Change doesn't happen overnight. It happens in the SMALL MOMENTS—the QUIET DECISIONS that shape your habits over time. That's why this book focuses on REALISTIC STRATEGIES that honor your BODY'S RHYTHMS and work with, not against, your NATURAL BIOLOGY.

You'll learn how to:

- REBUILD HORMONAL BALANCE by working with your body's natural cycles.
- INTERRUPT STRESS LOOPS before they spiral out of control.
- Create MICRO-HABITS that compound into LASTING TRANSFORMATION.
- Use SELF-AWARENESS to identify triggers and RESET YOUR MINDSET.
- Build CONNECTIONS and RITUALS that support long-term WELLNESS.

This isn't just about stress reduction. It's about EMPOWERMENT. When you learn to WORK WITH YOUR BODY, you step into a space of CONTROL—not by ELIMINATING STRESS entirely, but by MASTERING YOUR RESPONSE to it.

WHY NOW IS THE TIME TO TAKE BACK CONTROL

Stress has a way of CONVINCING US that we're TOO BUSY to slow down, TOO OVERWHELMED to make changes, and TOO FAR GONE to reset. But here's the truth—change starts the moment you DECIDE TO SHOW UP for yourself.

There's no PERFECT TIMING. There's only RIGHT NOW.

You don't have to wait for a CRISIS to hit before prioritizing BALANCE. By starting today, you're not just investing in STRESS RELIEF. You're investing in LONGEVITY, CLARITY, and the freedom to live with INTENTION.

MOVING FORWARD—ONE STEP AT A TIME

This book is your ROADMAP—not a RIGID SET OF RULES, but a GUIDE TO HELP YOU NAVIGATE the journey toward CALM, CLARITY, and RESILIENCE. Each chapter will help you DEEPEN YOUR UNDERSTANDING, EXPERIMENT WITH NEW PRACTICES, and FINE-TUNE YOUR APPROACH.

You're not just detoxing stress. You're RECLAIMING YOUR PEACE. And by the time you reach the final page, you won't just feel LIGHTER—you'll feel STRONGER, STEADIER, and more connected to YOURSELF than ever before.

Let's get started.

CHAPTER 1: UNDERSTANDING CORTISOL

Cortisol—often called the "stress hormone"—is one of the most influential chemicals in your body. It acts as a biological alarm system, responding to stress and regulating essential functions like energy production, metabolism, and immune response. But when cortisol levels become imbalanced, whether too high or too low, it can wreak havoc on both your physical and emotional health.

In today's fast-paced world, chronic stress has turned cortisol into a double-edged sword. Instead of providing short-term energy boosts and focus during moments of tension, excessive cortisol leaves many people fatigued, anxious, and struggling with weight gain. On the other hand, insufficient cortisol can lead to lethargy, apathy, and a weakened immune system.

This chapter breaks down what cortisol is, why it's essential for survival, and how modern habits can throw it out of balance. It examines symptoms of imbalance, the triggers behind these disruptions, and practical ways to test and monitor cortisol levels. Finally, it explores the importance of a cortisol detox—a targeted approach to reset your hormones, improve resilience, and restore well-being. Understanding cortisol is the first step toward reclaiming energy, focus, and calm in a chaotic world.

1.1 WHAT IS CORTISOL AND WHY IS IT IMPORTANT?

THE "ENGINE" OF YOUR BODY: WHY CORTISOL IS CRUCIAL

Cortisol is often referred to as the body's engine oil, an essential hormone that keeps your internal systems running smoothly. Produced by the adrenal glands, cortisol plays a pivotal role in your daily survival and well-being. While its reputation as the "stress hormone" is well-known, cortisol is much more than a mere byproduct of your stressful moments. It's a regulator, a balancer, and a key player in multiple physiological functions.

Think of cortisol as the ultimate multitasker. It helps regulate blood sugar levels, supports your metabolism, influences your immune responses, and even plays a role in memory formation. Without cortisol, your body's systems would operate like a machine without lubrication—grinding, inefficient, and prone to breakdowns.

At its core, cortisol works as part of the hypothalamic-pituitary-adrenal (HPA) axis, a sophisticated communication network between your brain and adrenal glands. This axis ensures cortisol is released in the right amounts at the right times. It's like a thermostat, maintaining a delicate balance to keep your body operating within optimal parameters.

CORTISOL AS THE "STRESS HORMONE"

While cortisol is vital for your health, its nickname as the "stress hormone" comes from its immediate response to perceived threats. Imagine you're crossing the street and a car unexpectedly speeds toward you. In a fraction of a second, your brain triggers the release of cortisol, preparing your body to fight or flee. Your heart rate accelerates, your blood pressure rises, and glucose floods into your bloodstream, giving you the energy to react swiftly.

This acute response is not just helpful—it's lifesaving. However, the challenge arises when stress becomes chronic. In today's world, where deadlines, notifications, and endless to-do lists dominate our days, the cortisol response can become overstimulated. Instead of functioning as a short-term lifesaver, it turns into a long-term saboteur, keeping your body in a state of heightened alert.

It's crucial to note that cortisol itself isn't the villain. The problem lies in its overproduction or mismanagement due to the demands of modern life. When cortisol remains elevated for prolonged periods, it can lead to a cascade of health issues, from disrupted sleep to impaired immunity.

THE MODERN LIFESTYLE AND ITS IMPACT ON CORTISOL BALANCE

Modern living is a double-edged sword. While technological advancements have made life more convenient, they've also introduced a new wave of stressors that our ancestors never faced. Email inboxes, social media comparisons, and the constant pressure to perform have created an environment where our bodies perceive danger around every corner—even if the threat is a mere work deadline.

This constant activation of the HPA axis causes cortisol to remain elevated, leading to a phenomenon often referred to as CORTISOL OVERLOAD. Our bodies were designed to handle short bursts of stress, but the chronic, low-level stressors of modern life disrupt this natural rhythm.

For instance, the blue light emitted by smartphones and laptops interferes with the production of melatonin, your sleep hormone, indirectly affecting cortisol's natural cycle. Instead of decreasing at night to allow for restful sleep, cortisol can remain elevated, leading to insomnia and restless nights. Similarly, skipping meals or relying on caffeine for energy spikes blood sugar levels, which in turn triggers cortisol production to stabilize your system.

THE ROLE OF CORTISOL IN YOUR BODY'S FUNCTIONS

Cortisol's impact extends far beyond stress. It is intricately woven into nearly every system in your body, making its regulation essential for overall health.

1. **Energy Management:** Cortisol ensures your body has enough energy to meet its demands. It does this by influencing how your body uses carbohydrates, fats, and proteins. For example, when blood sugar levels drop, cortisol helps release stored glucose into the bloodstream, maintaining steady energy levels.
2. **Inflammation and Immunity:** While acute cortisol spikes can suppress inflammation during injuries or illnesses, chronic elevation can weaken your immune system, making you more susceptible to infections.
3. **Mental Clarity:** Have you ever felt foggy or scatterbrained during stressful times? That's cortisol at play. While short-term cortisol boosts can sharpen focus and memory, prolonged exposure can impair cognitive function, particularly in areas of the brain like the hippocampus.
4. **Blood Pressure Regulation:** Cortisol helps maintain cardiovascular health by regulating blood pressure. However, when levels are consistently high, it can lead to hypertension and increase the risk of heart disease.
5. **Mood Regulation:** Cortisol also interacts with neurotransmitters like serotonin and dopamine, which influence mood. Imbalanced cortisol levels can contribute to feelings of anxiety, irritability, and even depression.

HOW CHRONIC STRESS AFFECTS YOUR HEALTH

When stress becomes a constant companion, the resulting cortisol dysregulation can create a domino effect on your physical and mental health. Chronic stress leads to a condition known as HPA AXIS DYSREGULATION, where the body struggles to maintain the appropriate cortisol balance.

1. **Weight Gain and Fatigue:** Elevated cortisol encourages fat storage, particularly around the abdomen, as a survival mechanism. This "stress belly" is not just a cosmetic concern—it's a risk factor for metabolic disorders. Simultaneously, chronic cortisol depletes your body's energy reserves, leaving you feeling perpetually tired.
2. **Disrupted Sleep Patterns:** High cortisol levels at night interfere with the body's natural ability to wind down, leading to insomnia or poor-quality sleep. Over time, this lack of rest further exacerbates cortisol imbalance, creating a vicious cycle.
3. **Weakened Immune System:** Constant cortisol elevation suppresses immune responses, making you more vulnerable to colds, infections, and even slower recovery from illnesses.
4. **Cognitive Decline:** Prolonged exposure to high cortisol can shrink the hippocampus, the brain region responsible for memory and learning. This can result in difficulty concentrating, forgetfulness, and mental fatigue.
5. **Mood Disorders:** Chronic cortisol dysregulation is often linked to anxiety and depression, as it disrupts the brain's chemical balance.

Cortisol is a hormone that exemplifies the importance of balance. While it serves as a critical component of survival and daily functioning, its overproduction—largely driven by the demands of modern living—can wreak havoc on your health. Understanding cortisol is the first step toward reclaiming control and achieving equilibrium in your body and mind.

1.2 SIGNS AND CAUSES OF CORTISOL IMBALANCE

TRIGGERS OF CORTISOL DYSREGULATION: POOR DIET, SLEEP DEPRIVATION, CHRONIC STRESS

Cortisol imbalance often begins as a silent disruption, quietly altering the body's internal rhythm before noticeable symptoms emerge. At the heart of this imbalance are MODERN LIFESTYLE FACTORS that place relentless demands on the body's stress response system. Poor diet, lack of sleep, and chronic stress are the three primary culprits responsible for pushing cortisol levels out of sync.

Dietary choices play a surprisingly influential role in cortisol regulation. Diets high in refined sugars, processed foods, and unhealthy fats spike blood sugar levels, forcing the body to release more cortisol to stabilize glucose. Similarly, skipping meals or consuming caffeine excessively can stimulate cortisol production as the body perceives hunger or overstimulation as a form of stress. In contrast, nutrient-dense diets rich in HEALTHY FATS, PROTEINS, AND COMPLEX CARBOHYDRATES help stabilize energy levels and reduce unnecessary cortisol spikes.

Sleep deprivation is another major driver of cortisol imbalance. Cortisol levels naturally follow a circadian rhythm, peaking in the morning to provide energy and gradually declining at night to prepare the body for rest. Poor sleep habits—whether caused by irregular sleep schedules, insomnia, or nighttime disruptions—interrupt this rhythm, often leading to ELEVATED NIGHTTIME CORTISOL. Over time, this pattern creates fatigue during the day and hyperactivity at night, leaving the body in a constant state of disarray.

Chronic stress, perhaps the most well-known trigger, keeps the adrenal glands in overdrive. Unlike acute stress, which resolves quickly, chronic stress forces the body to release cortisol continuously, exhausting the adrenal glands. This state of prolonged activation often stems from WORK PRESSURE, FINANCIAL WORRIES, EMOTIONAL STRUGGLES, or even unresolved trauma. The body interprets these stressors as ongoing threats, never receiving the signal to stand down and return to balance.

Together, these triggers create a cycle of CORTISOL DYSREGULATION that can spiral into more serious health issues if left unaddressed. Identifying these triggers is the first step toward breaking the cycle and restoring hormonal balance.

SYMPTOMS OF HIGH CORTISOL: ANXIETY, WEIGHT GAIN, INSOMNIA, FATIGUE

When cortisol levels remain elevated for extended periods, the effects ripple across multiple systems in the body. The symptoms of HIGH CORTISOL are often subtle at first, but over time, they can intensify and disrupt daily life.

1. **Anxiety and Irritability:** One of the most immediate effects of high cortisol is an increase in feelings of anxiety, nervousness, and irritability. Elevated cortisol enhances alertness, but when sustained, it can lead to HYPERVIGILANCE, making it difficult to relax or focus.

2. **Weight Gain, Particularly Around the Abdomen:** High cortisol levels prompt the body to store fat—especially around the midsection—as a protective mechanism. This type of fat storage, known as VISCERAL FAT, is not only stubborn but also metabolically active, increasing inflammation and raising the risk of cardiovascular disease.

3. **Insomnia and Restlessness:** Persistent cortisol spikes interfere with the body's ability to wind down at night. This leads to DIFFICULTY FALLING ASLEEP, STAYING ASLEEP, OR FEELING RESTED in the morning. Over time, poor sleep worsens cortisol dysregulation, creating a vicious cycle.

4. **Fatigue Despite High Energy Spikes:** Many people with high cortisol levels report feeling WIRED BUT TIRED—mentally alert but physically exhausted. This paradox occurs because cortisol forces the body into a state of high alert, depleting energy reserves without allowing adequate recovery.

5. **Digestive Issues:** High cortisol diverts blood flow away from the digestive system, leading to BLOATING, INDIGESTION, AND IRREGULAR BOWEL MOVEMENTS. Chronic stress can also reduce the production of stomach acid, impairing nutrient absorption.
6. **Frequent Illness and Infections:** Cortisol suppresses immune function in the short term, which is beneficial during acute stress. However, chronic elevation can WEAKEN IMMUNITY, leaving the body vulnerable to frequent colds, infections, and inflammation.

Recognizing these symptoms early allows individuals to take corrective action before the imbalance becomes more deeply ingrained.

SYMPTOMS OF LOW CORTISOL: CHRONIC FATIGUE, APATHY, LACK OF ENERGY

While high cortisol gets most of the attention, LOW CORTISOL—a state often caused by adrenal fatigue—can be equally disruptive. After prolonged overproduction, the adrenal glands may eventually burn out, leading to a state where the body struggles to produce adequate cortisol. This condition, sometimes referred to as ADRENAL INSUFFICIENCY, brings its own set of challenges.

1. **Chronic Fatigue and Exhaustion:** Unlike the jittery fatigue associated with high cortisol, low cortisol causes DEEP, UNRELENTING TIREDNESS. People with low cortisol often feel exhausted even after a full night's sleep.
2. **Apathy and Low Motivation:** Cortisol plays a key role in ENERGY MOBILIZATION and motivation. When levels drop too low, it can lead to feelings of apathy, disinterest, and emotional flatness. Tasks that once felt manageable may suddenly feel overwhelming.
3. **Brain Fog and Poor Concentration:** Low cortisol reduces blood sugar levels, depriving the brain of glucose and resulting in MENTAL FOGGINESS, FORGETFULNESS, and difficulty processing information.
4. **Muscle Weakness and Joint Pain:** Cortisol supports muscle and joint health by reducing inflammation. Insufficient levels can lead to STIFFNESS, SORENESS, and a general sense of physical weakness.
5. **Low Blood Pressure and Dizziness:** Without enough cortisol to regulate vascular tone, some individuals may experience DIZZINESS, LIGHTHEADEDNESS, or even fainting, particularly when standing up quickly.
6. **Cravings for Salt and Sugar:** The body may compensate for low cortisol by craving SALTY AND SUGARY FOODS to help stabilize blood pressure and energy levels. While these cravings provide temporary relief, they often lead to further imbalances.

THE IMPORTANCE OF RECOGNIZING EARLY WARNING SIGNS

Cortisol imbalance doesn't happen overnight. It often begins with mild symptoms—occasional fatigue, irritability, or difficulty sleeping—that are easy to dismiss. Over time, these early signs can snowball into chronic conditions that affect mental, emotional, and physical well-being.

Paying attention to PATTERNS AND CHANGES in your body is crucial. For instance, consistently waking up tired despite a full night's rest may indicate elevated nighttime cortisol. On the other hand, struggling to get out of bed in the morning may signal low cortisol.

Equally important is acknowledging the emotional and psychological impacts. Persistent feelings of anxiety, sadness, or lack of motivation are often tied to hormonal imbalances, even when they don't present obvious physical symptoms.

By identifying triggers and recognizing symptoms early, individuals can take proactive steps to support adrenal health and restore cortisol balance before the effects become debilitating.

1.3 HOW TO TEST AND MONITOR CORTISOL LEVELS

Understanding how to measure cortisol levels is essential for identifying imbalances and taking proactive steps toward restoring hormonal health. Testing provides a SNAPSHOT of your body's stress response and helps uncover whether cortisol levels are too high, too low, or fluctuating irregularly throughout the day.

Cortisol testing is not a one-size-fits-all process. Different methods capture unique aspects of cortisol behavior, from MOMENTARY SPIKES to LONG-TERM PATTERNS. Choosing the right test and interpreting the results can be the key to addressing adrenal health effectively.

LAB TESTS: SALIVA, BLOOD, AND URINE – WHICH WORKS BEST?

Testing cortisol levels involves evaluating how your body produces and regulates this critical hormone. Each testing method has its strengths, and understanding them helps determine the most accurate approach for your specific needs.

SALIVA TESTING: CAPTURING DAILY PATTERNS

Saliva tests are widely regarded as one of the most convenient and effective methods for measuring cortisol. These tests focus on FREE CORTISOL—the active form of the hormone available to tissues—and can track how levels fluctuate throughout the day.

Because cortisol naturally follows a DIURNAL RHYTHM, saliva testing is often conducted multiple times a day—morning, noon, evening, and night—to assess these variations. Elevated readings at night, for example, might explain INSOMNIA OR NIGHTTIME ANXIETY. Low readings in the morning could point to ADRENAL FATIGUE and a sluggish stress response.

Advantages of Saliva Testing:

- **Non-invasive:** Collecting saliva samples is painless and easy, making it ideal for at-home use.
- **Captures fluctuations:** Multiple samples throughout the day reveal CIRCADIAN RHYTHMS and patterns.
- **Accurate for free cortisol:** Reflects bioavailable cortisol, the type your body actively uses.

Limitations:

- Less effective for measuring TOTAL CORTISOL OUTPUT.
- May not detect rare adrenal disorders, such as Addison's or Cushing's disease.

BLOOD TESTING: MEASURING BOUND CORTISOL

Blood tests, or SERUM CORTISOL TESTS, are commonly used in clinical settings to measure cortisol levels. Unlike saliva tests, they assess TOTAL CORTISOL, which includes both free cortisol and cortisol bound to proteins.

Because cortisol spikes under stress, even the act of drawing blood can trigger a rise in levels, potentially skewing results. For this reason, blood tests often provide a SINGLE SNAPSHOT rather than capturing the fluctuations that occur throughout the day.

Advantages of Blood Testing:

- **Widely available:** Most healthcare providers offer this test.
- **Helpful for diagnosing adrenal disorders:** Can identify conditions like CUSHING'S SYNDROME and ADDISON'S DISEASE.

Limitations:

- **Stress-sensitive:** The testing process itself may artificially elevate cortisol.
- **Limited timing:** A single measurement may not reflect DAILY PATTERNS or CHRONIC IMBALANCES.

URINE TESTING: ASSESSING LONG-TERM OUTPUT

Urine tests measure METABOLIZED CORTISOL, providing a broader picture of hormone production over time. These tests are particularly useful for identifying CORTISOL METABOLITES—the breakdown products of cortisol—which can reveal how efficiently the body processes the hormone.

Most urine tests require 24-hour collection, capturing total cortisol output rather than momentary spikes. This method is especially helpful for uncovering HIDDEN IMBALANCES that may not be obvious with saliva or blood tests.

Advantages of Urine Testing:
- **Comprehensive data:** Measures both free and metabolized cortisol for a fuller picture.
- **Detects patterns over time:** Reflects long-term trends rather than momentary fluctuations.

Limitations:
- **Less convenient:** Requires collecting and storing urine samples over 24 hours.
- **Limited insight into daily rhythms:** Doesn't capture TIME-SPECIFIC SPIKES OR DIPS.

AT-HOME TESTING KITS: ACCURACY AND CONVENIENCE

At-home cortisol testing kits have surged in popularity, offering an accessible way to monitor hormone health without visiting a doctor's office. Most kits rely on SALIVA or URINE SAMPLES and are designed to detect patterns associated with adrenal dysfunction.

Ease of Use: Modern kits provide detailed instructions for sample collection, allowing users to track cortisol at multiple times of day or over a 24-hour period. These kits often include pre-paid mailers to send samples to certified labs, making the process simple and discreet.

Reliability and Accuracy: While at-home tests are highly accurate for ROUTINE MONITORING, they may lack the precision needed for diagnosing complex disorders like ADRENAL INSUFFICIENCY or CUSHING'S SYNDROME. In such cases, laboratory testing is often recommended as a follow-up.

Key Features of At-Home Kits:
- **Multi-sample collection:** Tracks fluctuations over time.
- **Detailed reports:** Provides data on trends and rhythms.
- **Affordable and accessible:** Eliminates the need for clinical appointments.

UNDERSTANDING YOUR RESULTS: WHEN TO TAKE ACTION

Interpreting cortisol test results requires looking beyond the numbers to understand how they correlate with symptoms and lifestyle factors. Normal cortisol patterns follow a CURVE—high in the morning, tapering off throughout the day, and hitting their lowest point at night.

WHAT HIGH CORTISOL MEANS

Elevated readings often point to CHRONIC STRESS, INFLAMMATION, or adrenal overactivity. Key signs include:
- Persistent fatigue despite adequate sleep.
- Difficulty relaxing or feeling "on edge."
- WEIGHT GAIN, especially around the abdomen.

High cortisol may also suggest HIDDEN STRESSORS, such as blood sugar imbalances, sleep disturbances, or underlying infections that trigger inflammation.

WHAT LOW CORTISOL MEANS

Low readings often signal ADRENAL FATIGUE or burnout, where the glands can no longer sustain cortisol production. Symptoms include:
- EXHAUSTION, even after rest.
- Low motivation or feelings of apathy.
- Cravings for SALTY FOODS.

Low cortisol levels can also be associated with IMMUNE SUPPRESSION, making the body more vulnerable to infections and prolonged recovery periods.

RECOGNIZING PATTERNS, NOT JUST NUMBERS

Testing cortisol isn't about chasing the "perfect" number. It's about identifying PATTERNS—how cortisol behaves over the course of the day and how it responds to stress.

For instance, HIGH MORNING CORTISOL paired with LOW EVENING LEVELS might indicate EARLY-STAGE ADRENAL DYSFUNCTION. Conversely, FLATLINED CORTISOL CURVES could point to advanced ADRENAL BURNOUT.

Tracking these trends helps individuals and healthcare providers develop personalized strategies, whether through DIETARY ADJUSTMENTS, STRESS REDUCTION TECHNIQUES, or targeted supplements.

WHEN TESTING BECOMES ESSENTIAL

Routine cortisol testing is especially valuable for individuals experiencing:

- UNEXPLAINED FATIGUE that doesn't improve with rest.
- SUDDEN WEIGHT GAIN OR LOSS.
- PERSISTENT INSOMNIA or disrupted sleep cycles.
- MOOD SWINGS, ANXIETY, or brain fog.

Early detection not only reveals underlying imbalances but also allows for PREVENTATIVE MEASURES before symptoms escalate into chronic conditions.

Monitoring cortisol levels empowers individuals to take control of their health, paving the way for RESTORATION, BALANCE, and lasting wellness.

1.4 WHY DO A CORTISOL DETOX?

Cortisol plays a central role in maintaining BALANCE in the body, but when it spirals out of control, it can leave you feeling TIRED, OVERWHELMED, and physically unwell. A CORTISOL DETOX offers a way to reset your stress hormones, helping your body regain its NATURAL RHYTHM and function more effectively.

This process isn't just about eliminating toxins—it's about restoring harmony to your endocrine system and teaching your body how to ADAPT to stress without triggering a hormonal firestorm.

THE NEGATIVE EFFECTS OF CORTISOL OVERLOAD

When cortisol remains elevated for too long, it starts to work AGAINST your body instead of supporting it. Chronic stress can trick your adrenal glands into releasing cortisol NON-STOP, leading to HORMONAL CHAOS.

DISRUPTED SLEEP PATTERNS

One of the first casualties of high cortisol is SLEEP. Normally, cortisol levels should drop at night, signaling your body to wind down. But when cortisol stays high, your body gets stuck in "ALERT MODE", making it difficult to relax.

- **Struggling to fall asleep** becomes a nightly battle.
- **Frequent wake-ups** leave you feeling unrested.
- **Morning fatigue** persists, no matter how many hours you spend in bed.

Over time, poor sleep can lead to MEMORY ISSUES, IRRITABILITY, and weakened IMMUNITY.

WEIGHT GAIN AND CRAVINGS

Cortisol is deeply connected to METABOLISM. When it's elevated, your body starts storing FAT, especially around the abdomen. This VISCERAL FAT is not only hard to shed but also increases the risk of DIABETES AND HEART DISEASE.

Additionally, cortisol spikes cause BLOOD SUGAR FLUCTUATIONS, triggering INTENSE CRAVINGS for sugary or fatty foods. These cravings are your body's attempt to replenish ENERGY RESERVES quickly—but they often lead to WEIGHT GAIN.

FATIGUE AND ENERGY CRASHES

Paradoxically, even though high cortisol keeps you WIRED, it also leaves you WORN OUT. Your adrenal glands eventually become OVERWORKED, struggling to keep up with constant demands.

- ENERGY CRASHES hit suddenly, leaving you drained.
- Even after resting, you may feel LETHARGIC and unmotivated.

This rollercoaster effect can make it impossible to maintain CONSISTENT ENERGY LEVELS.

MOOD SWINGS AND ANXIETY

Cortisol has a direct impact on MOOD REGULATION. Excess cortisol interferes with SEROTONIN and DOPAMINE production—the brain chemicals responsible for HAPPINESS AND RELAXATION.

- Increased ANXIETY leaves you feeling on edge.
- Irritability and MOOD SWINGS become common.
- Difficulty concentrating leads to BRAIN FOG.

Over time, this hormonal imbalance can even contribute to DEPRESSION.

THE BENEFITS OF A DETOX: RECLAIMING BALANCE

A cortisol detox is designed to INTERRUPT these harmful cycles and create a foundation for LASTING WELLNESS. By reducing triggers, calming the nervous system, and supporting adrenal health, this process helps the body RESET.

IMPROVED SLEEP QUALITY

Balancing cortisol levels allows your body to reestablish a HEALTHY CIRCADIAN RHYTHM. As cortisol drops in the evening, melatonin—the SLEEP HORMONE—rises naturally.

- Falling asleep becomes EASIER.
- Sleep cycles become DEEPER and more restorative.
- Waking up feels REFRESHING instead of exhausting.

Many people who complete a cortisol detox report waking up with a sense of CLARITY and FOCUS they haven't experienced in years.

STEADY ENERGY THROUGHOUT THE DAY

Resetting cortisol levels helps smooth out ENERGY FLUCTUATIONS. Instead of feeling WIRED AND TIRED, you experience SUSTAINED ENERGY.

- Midday crashes become RARE.
- Focus and MENTAL CLARITY improve.
- The body uses ENERGY MORE EFFICIENTLY.

This shift allows you to STAY PRODUCTIVE without relying on caffeine or sugar for quick boosts.

WEIGHT LOSS AND BETTER METABOLISM

Once cortisol levels stabilize, your body becomes more RESPONSIVE to diet and exercise. Instead of holding onto FAT STORES, it shifts back to BURNING CALORIES efficiently.

- Belly fat diminishes as INFLAMMATION SUBSIDES.
- Blood sugar stabilizes, reducing CRAVINGS.
- Digestion improves, supporting NUTRIENT ABSORPTION.

These metabolic changes make it easier to maintain a HEALTHY WEIGHT.

REDUCED ANXIETY AND EMOTIONAL STABILITY

A cortisol detox not only calms the ADRENAL GLANDS but also soothes the NERVOUS SYSTEM. Stress responses become more MEASURED, leaving you feeling GROUNDED instead of overwhelmed.

- Anxiety levels decrease as CORTISOL RECEPTORS RESET.
- Mood swings give way to EMOTIONAL BALANCE.
- Increased SEROTONIN AND DOPAMINE levels promote a sense of WELL-BEING.

This newfound EMOTIONAL STABILITY makes it easier to handle life's challenges without feeling OVERWHELMED.

HOW THIS DETOX CAN TRANSFORM YOUR LIFE

A cortisol detox isn't a QUICK FIX—it's a comprehensive approach to REWIRING your body's response to stress. It goes beyond temporary relief, creating LONG-TERM RESILIENCE against modern stressors.

RESTORING HORMONAL HARMONY

The detox process focuses on giving the adrenal glands time to RECOVER. It involves:

- Nourishing the body with ANTI-INFLAMMATORY FOODS.
- Eliminating STIMULANTS like caffeine that keep cortisol high.
- Incorporating ADAPTOGENS—herbs that support adrenal health.

By addressing NUTRITIONAL GAPS and removing triggers, the adrenal system can HEAL and regain balance.

ENHANCING STRESS RESILIENCE

Detoxing from cortisol overload also strengthens your MENTAL RESILIENCE. Mindfulness practices, such as MEDITATION AND YOGA, retrain the brain to handle stress without triggering HORMONAL SURGES.

These habits not only REDUCE STRESS HORMONES but also build EMOTIONAL STRENGTH to face future challenges.

SUPPORTING LONG-TERM HEALTH

Perhaps the greatest benefit of a cortisol detox is the impact on LONGEVITY. By preventing the damaging effects of CHRONIC INFLAMMATION, you reduce the risk of:

- HEART DISEASE.
- DIABETES.
- COGNITIVE DECLINE.

This approach shifts the focus from SYMPTOM MANAGEMENT to LASTING VITALITY.

A HOLISTIC APPROACH TO HEALING

A cortisol detox isn't just about addressing PHYSICAL SYMPTOMS—it's about transforming your relationship with STRESS. By resetting your HORMONAL RHYTHMS, you're giving your body the tools it needs to thrive in an OVERSTIMULATED WORLD.

Whether you're battling FATIGUE, WEIGHT GAIN, or ANXIETY, this process creates a foundation for LASTING CHANGE. Instead of simply surviving, you regain the ability to THRIVE—mentally, physically, and emotionally.

Conclusion to Chapter 1: Understanding Cortisol

Cortisol is not the ENEMY—it's a VITAL HORMONE that powers ENERGY, IMMUNITY, and ADAPTABILITY to stress. But IMBALANCED CORTISOL can trigger HEALTH PROBLEMS. Knowing the SIGNS OF DYSREGULATION and how to TEST your levels gives you control over your HEALTH JOURNEY.

A CORTISOL DETOX helps RESET hormonal rhythms, ease OVERWORKED ADRENALS, and restore CALM AND BALANCE. It's about building RESILIENCE—physically, mentally, and emotionally. With these insights, you're ready to take the first steps toward HEALING and LONG-TERM WELLNESS.

CHAPTER 2: THE FOUNDATIONS OF CORTISOL DETOX

Modern life often demands more than our bodies are naturally equipped to handle. Deadlines, screens, late nights, and processed foods create an endless cycle of *stress triggers* that keep cortisol levels *elevated*. Over time, this hormonal imbalance erodes our *energy*, disrupts *sleep patterns*, and leaves us feeling *fatigued* and *overwhelmed*. Rebalancing cortisol isn't just about addressing the symptoms—it's about resetting the *foundation* of how your body handles stress.

This chapter introduces the *building blocks* of a successful cortisol detox, focusing on *holistic strategies* that address the root causes of imbalance. These foundations aren't quick fixes; they are *sustainable practices* designed to *nurture hormonal health* and restore *calm* to your mind and body. From *nutrition* and *natural remedies* to *mindfulness practices* and *circadian rhythm alignment*, each pillar plays a crucial role in *retraining your stress response*.

Think of this chapter as your *roadmap*—a step-by-step guide to creating an *environment* and *routine* that actively supports *hormonal balance*. Whether you're battling *burnout* or looking to *optimize wellness*, these nine pillars provide the *tools* you need to reclaim your *energy*, *focus*, and *inner calm*.

2.1 PREPARING FOR CHANGE

Transforming your health begins with PREPARATION. Before diving into a cortisol detox, it's critical to establish a BASELINE, identify STRESS TRIGGERS, and gather the TOOLS that will set you up for SUCCESS. Think of this phase as laying the FOUNDATION for a more BALANCED, RESILIENT, and ENERGIZED VERSION of yourself. When approached with INTENTION and CLARITY, preparation not only simplifies the process but also strengthens your COMMITMENT to long-term WELL-BEING.

MEASURING YOUR STRESS LEVELS: A SIMPLE STARTING POINT

Understanding where you STAND is the first step toward CHANGE. Stress affects everyone differently, and the DEGREE to which cortisol is DISRUPTED depends on factors like LIFESTYLE, GENETICS, and ENVIRONMENT. To PERSONALIZE your detox, you need to measure your STRESS RESPONSE and determine whether your cortisol is OVERACTIVE, UNDERACTIVE, or fluctuating between the two.

SELF-ASSESSMENT TOOLS

Begin with a SELF-ASSESSMENT QUESTIONNAIRE. Reflect on the following questions:

- Do you wake up feeling EXHAUSTED, even after a full night's sleep?
- Are you experiencing FREQUENT CRAVINGS for SALTY or SUGARY foods?
- Do you find yourself IRRITABLE, ANXIOUS, or prone to MOOD SWINGS?
- Have you noticed UNEXPLAINED WEIGHT GAIN, particularly around your MIDSECTION?
- Are your energy levels INCONSISTENT, with periods of HIGH ENERGY followed by CRASHES?
- Do you experience BRAIN FOG or difficulty CONCENTRATING?

Your answers provide a SNAPSHOT of your CURRENT STATE. If multiple symptoms resonate, it's a sign your CORTISOL LEVELS may be OUT OF BALANCE.

TRACKING PATTERNS

Keep a STRESS JOURNAL for at least THREE TO FIVE DAYS. Record:

- WHAT triggered your stress (work deadlines, social pressures, poor sleep)?
- HOW your body responded (headaches, fatigue, tension)?
- The TIME OF DAY symptoms occurred.

Recognizing PATTERNS can reveal HIDDEN TRIGGERS—whether it's a LATE-NIGHT SNACK disrupting your SLEEP CYCLE or a LACK OF DOWNTIME leaving you perpetually ON EDGE.

ESSENTIAL TOOLS FOR SUCCESS: JOURNALS, PLANNERS, AND BASIC INGREDIENTS

A CORTISOL DETOX isn't just about REMOVING TOXINS. It's about creating a STRUCTURED FRAMEWORK for HEALING and REBALANCING your body. Having the right TOOLS can make the process MANAGEABLE, MOTIVATING, and REWARDING.

THE POWER OF JOURNALING

A WELL-KEPT JOURNAL serves as both a TRACKER and a THERAPEUTIC OUTLET. Use it to:

- Log DAILY MEALS, WATER INTAKE, and SUPPLEMENTS.
- Monitor ENERGY LEVELS and MOOD FLUCTUATIONS.
- Reflect on EMOTIONAL TRIGGERS and WINS.

Writing things down not only creates ACCOUNTABILITY but also helps you CONNECT THE DOTS between habits and HORMONAL HEALTH.

PLANNERS AND CALENDARS

Consistency is KEY. Organize your SCHEDULE to include:

- MEAL PREP days for stress-reducing foods.
- Time slots for EXERCISE, MEDITATION, and SLEEP HYGIENE.
- Reminders to HYDRATE and TAKE SUPPLEMENTS.

A planner transforms VAGUE INTENTIONS into ACTIONABLE STEPS.

CORE INGREDIENTS FOR DETOX SUPPORT

Stock your kitchen with WHOLE FOODS rich in MAGNESIUM, B VITAMINS, and HEALTHY FATS—nutrients that NOURISH ADRENAL GLANDS and STABILIZE BLOOD SUGAR. Essential items include:

- LEAFY GREENS (spinach, kale) for MAGNESIUM.
- FATTY FISH (salmon, mackerel) for OMEGA-3S.
- SEEDS and NUTS (chia, almonds) for ZINC and ANTIOXIDANTS.
- HERBAL TEAS like ASHWAGANDHA and HOLY BASIL to promote CALM.

Keeping your pantry STOCKED eliminates the temptation for PROCESSED SNACKS and CAFFEINE OVERLOAD.

TAKING THE INITIAL TEST: UNDERSTANDING YOUR CURRENT STATE

A CLINICAL TEST provides DATA-DRIVEN INSIGHTS into your CORTISOL PROFILE. While self-assessments offer CLUES, lab tests pinpoint BIOCHEMICAL IMBALANCES.

TYPES OF CORTISOL TESTS

1. **Saliva Tests** – Measure CORTISOL FLUCTUATIONS throughout the day. Ideal for assessing CIRCADIAN RHYTHM DISRUPTIONS.
2. **Blood Tests** – Offer a SINGLE-POINT SNAPSHOT. Best for measuring BASAL CORTISOL LEVELS.
3. **Urine Tests** – Analyze METABOLIZED CORTISOL. Useful for identifying LONG-TERM PATTERNS.

TIMING MATTERS

Cortisol naturally follows a DIURNAL RHYTHM, peaking in the MORNING and tapering off by EVENING. Testing at the WRONG TIME can produce MISLEADING RESULTS.

For saliva tests, aim for:

- **Morning sample** (30 minutes after waking) to assess your BASELINE SURGE.
- **Afternoon sample** to check for STRESS BUILDUP.
- **Evening sample** to measure WIND-DOWN CAPACITY.

AT-HOME KITS VS. LAB TESTING
At-home kits are convenient and allow for multiple samples across the day, but laboratory testing provides comprehensive PANELS. Discuss results with a HEALTHCARE PROVIDER to ensure ACCURATE INTERPRETATIONS.

BUILDING YOUR FOUNDATION FOR CHANGE
The DETOX JOURNEY starts with AWARENESS. By measuring your STRESS LOAD, assembling TOOLS FOR SUCCESS, and taking TESTS to map out your CORTISOL RHYTHMS, you lay the groundwork for TRANSFORMATION. Preparation isn't just about PLANNING MEALS or BUYING SUPPLEMENTS—it's about building a SYSTEM that supports CONSISTENCY, GROWTH, and ACCOUNTABILITY.

Approach this phase with CURIOSITY and OPENNESS. The insights you gain now will help you CUSTOMIZE your approach, STREAMLINE OBSTACLES, and focus on WHAT TRULY MATTERS: reclaiming your ENERGY, MENTAL CLARITY, and EMOTIONAL RESILIENCE.

2.2 THE NINE PILLARS OF CORTISOL DETOX
Rebalancing cortisol isn't about quick fixes or temporary solutions. It's about creating a SUSTAINABLE LIFESTYLE that nurtures both BODY and MIND. This process requires attention to the FUNDAMENTAL PILLARS of health—those core elements that influence how your HORMONES FUNCTION, how your NERVOUS SYSTEM REGULATES STRESS, and how your ENERGY LEVELS remain stable throughout the day.

These NINE PILLARS OF CORTISOL DETOX form the foundation of a TARGETED APPROACH designed to reset your CORTISOL RHYTHMS, promote HORMONAL HARMONY, and rebuild RESILIENCE against daily stressors. Each pillar contributes to your ability to MANAGE STRESS, RESTORE BALANCE, and PROTECT YOUR LONG-TERM WELL-BEING.

1. NUTRITION: FOODS THAT HELP REGULATE CORTISOL
CORTISOL REGULATION begins in the KITCHEN. The foods you eat play a DIRECT ROLE in stabilizing BLOOD SUGAR LEVELS, reducing INFLAMMATION, and supplying the NUTRIENTS your adrenal glands need to function optimally.

ANTI-INFLAMMATORY FOODS
Chronic stress often triggers INFLAMMATION, which exacerbates HORMONAL IMBALANCES. Incorporating ANTI-INFLAMMATORY FOODS like LEAFY GREENS, BERRIES, FATTY FISH, and TURMERIC helps NEUTRALIZE FREE RADICALS and REDUCE STRESS-INDUCED DAMAGE.

COMPLEX CARBOHYDRATES
WHOLE GRAINS, SWEET POTATOES, and LEGUMES provide SLOW-DIGESTING CARBOHYDRATES that PREVENT BLOOD SUGAR CRASHES. These crashes often signal your body to produce MORE CORTISOL in an attempt to compensate for the drop.

HEALTHY FATS
AVOCADOS, CHIA SEEDS, FLAXSEEDS, and OLIVE OIL support HORMONAL PRODUCTION and BRAIN HEALTH. They also aid in REDUCING INFLAMMATION and FUELING CELLULAR REPAIR.

PROTEIN-RICH FOODS
Lean proteins, such as CHICKEN, TURKEY, EGGS, and TOFU, are essential for AMINO ACID PRODUCTION. Amino acids like TYROSINE help create NEUROTRANSMITTERS that regulate MOOD and STRESS RESPONSES.

2. LIFESTYLE: SLEEP, MOVEMENT, AND STRESS MANAGEMENT
Lifestyle habits shape how your NERVOUS SYSTEM reacts to EXTERNAL PRESSURES. Three lifestyle factors—SLEEP, MOVEMENT, and STRESS MANAGEMENT—act as the CORNERSTONES for HORMONAL BALANCE.

PRIORITIZING SLEEP HYGIENE
CORTISOL LEVELS naturally drop in the EVENING, signaling your body to RELAX. Poor sleep habits disrupt this cycle, keeping cortisol levels ELEVATED. Focus on:
- CONSISTENT SLEEP SCHEDULES—going to bed and waking up at the SAME TIME.
- A COOL, DARK BEDROOM free of screens.

- WIND-DOWN ROUTINES that include READING, STRETCHING, or DEEP BREATHING.

MOVEMENT AND EXERCISE
- PHYSICAL ACTIVITY helps METABOLIZE EXCESS CORTISOL, but the TYPE and INTENSITY matter.
- GENTLE EXERCISES like YOGA, TAI CHI, and WALKING lower stress without overstimulating cortisol.
- STRENGTH TRAINING and CARDIO in MODERATE AMOUNTS boost ENDORPHINS but should be balanced to avoid overexertion.

STRESS-REDUCTION TECHNIQUES
Practices like PROGRESSIVE MUSCLE RELAXATION, BREATHWORK, and GUIDED IMAGERY help your nervous system shift into a PARASYMPATHETIC STATE—the mode where HEALING and RESTORATION occur.

3. NATURAL REMEDIES: ADAPTOGENS, AROMATHERAPY, AND SUPPLEMENTS
Nature offers POTENT ALLIES for cortisol regulation. ADAPTOGENS and ESSENTIAL OILS act as tools to NOURISH the ADRENAL GLANDS, while SUPPLEMENTS fill NUTRITIONAL GAPS.

ADAPTOGENIC HERBS
- ASHWAGANDHA reduces ANXIETY and stabilizes CORTISOL SPIKES.
- RHODIOLA enhances MENTAL FOCUS and PHYSICAL ENDURANCE.
- HOLY BASIL lowers BLOOD SUGAR and CALMS NERVES.

AROMATHERAPY
Essential oils like LAVENDER, BERGAMOT, and FRANKINCENSE promote RELAXATION and lower HEART RATE VARIABILITY, signaling a STRESS REDUCTION response.

KEY SUPPLEMENTS
- MAGNESIUM soothes MUSCLES and improves SLEEP.
- VITAMIN C supports ADRENAL FUNCTION.
- B VITAMINS aid in ENERGY METABOLISM and STRESS RECOVERY.

4. HYDRATION: THE IMPORTANCE OF FUNCTIONAL BEVERAGES
DEHYDRATION can ELEVATE CORTISOL LEVELS, amplifying the STRESS RESPONSE. Hydration goes beyond water—it includes MINERAL-RICH BEVERAGES that restore ELECTROLYTE BALANCE.

ELECTROLYTE-RICH DRINKS
Coconut water, BONE BROTH, and HOMEMADE ELECTROLYTE SOLUTIONS replenish MINERALS lost during STRESSFUL PERIODS.

HERBAL TEAS
- CHAMOMILE calms the NERVOUS SYSTEM.
- LEMON BALM reduces ANXIETY.
- LICORICE ROOT supports ADRENAL RECOVERY.

5. ENVIRONMENTAL CHANGES: CREATING A CALM LIVING SPACE
Your PHYSICAL SURROUNDINGS impact your MENTAL STATE. A CLUTTERED ENVIRONMENT can trigger MENTAL OVERWHELM, while a CALM SPACE encourages RELAXATION.

DECLUTTERING AND ORGANIZATION
- Simplify your WORKSPACE to reduce MENTAL NOISE.
- Incorporate SOOTHING COLORS like BLUE and GREEN.

NATURAL ELEMENTS
- Add PLANTS like PEACE LILIES or SNAKE PLANTS to PURIFY AIR and create VISUAL CALM.
- Maximize NATURAL LIGHT to support your CIRCADIAN RHYTHM.

6. CIRCADIAN RHYTHM: ALIGNING YOUR BODY CLOCK WITH NATURE

LIGHT EXPOSURE and DAILY ROUTINES influence CORTISOL PRODUCTION. Syncing your schedule with your INTERNAL CLOCK reduces HORMONAL MISALIGNMENT.

MORNING RITUALS
Expose yourself to NATURAL LIGHT within 30 MINUTES of waking to signal the brain to LOWER MELATONIN and BOOST CORTISOL.

EVENING WIND-DOWN
Dim lights at night and avoid SCREENS to help cortisol DECLINE NATURALLY.

7. MINDFULNESS PRACTICES: GRATITUDE, MEDITATION, AND JOURNALING

Practices that ANCHOR YOU IN THE PRESENT lower PERCEIVED STRESS and CALM OVERACTIVE CORTISOL RESPONSES.

- GRATITUDE JOURNALING shifts focus to POSITIVE EMOTIONS.
- MEDITATION quiets the MIND and lowers BLOOD PRESSURE.
- JOURNALING clarifies THOUGHTS and RELEASES TENSION.

8. NATURE CONNECTION: REAPING THE BENEFITS OF OUTDOOR ACTIVITIES

Spending time outdoors resets your NERVOUS SYSTEM. Nature exposure reduces STRESS HORMONES, boosts MOOD, and increases MENTAL CLARITY.

- FOREST BATHING improves HEART RATE VARIABILITY.
- WALKING BAREFOOT (grounding) stabilizes ELECTRICAL BALANCE.

9. PLAY AND CREATIVITY: THE STRESS-RELIEF POWER OF JOY

PLAY isn't just for kids—it's an ESSENTIAL TOOL for ADULTS to DEACTIVATE STRESS RESPONSES. Activities like PAINTING, DANCING, or GARDENING shift focus from PROBLEMS to PLEASURE, reducing CORTISOL BUILDUP.

These NINE PILLARS create a COMPREHENSIVE FRAMEWORK for restoring HORMONAL BALANCE and enhancing RESILIENCE.

Conclusion to Chapter 2: The Foundations of Cortisol Detox

Cortisol detox isn't just a process—it's a *lifestyle shift*. The nine pillars explored in this chapter work together to form a *comprehensive framework* for *stress recovery* and *hormonal balance*. By prioritizing *nourishing foods, restorative sleep, mindful practices,* and *natural remedies,* you're laying the groundwork for *lasting change*.

This journey isn't about perfection; it's about *consistency*. Small, intentional actions—like sipping a *calming herbal tea* or stepping outside for *fresh air*—can create *ripple effects* that transform how your body *processes stress*.

The foundation you're building here sets the stage for deeper healing in the chapters ahead. With each step, you're not only *lowering cortisol* but also *empowering yourself* to live with more *vitality, resilience,* and *peace*.

CHAPTER 3: THE DETOX NUTRITION PLAN

3.1 FOODS THAT HELP AND HURT CORTISOL LEVELS

Cortisol, often called the STRESS HORMONE, is deeply influenced by what we eat. Food is more than fuel—it's a MESSAGE to your body, telling it whether to prepare for stress or relax into recovery. The right foods can STABILIZE BLOOD SUGAR, REDUCE INFLAMMATION, and NOURISH ADRENAL GLANDS, helping to REGULATE CORTISOL PRODUCTION. On the other hand, poor dietary choices can SPIKE CORTISOL, leaving you feeling WIRED, TIRED, and OUT OF BALANCE.

This section explores the NUTRITIONAL STRATEGIES that support CORTISOL DETOXIFICATION by focusing on CORTISOL-FRIENDLY FOODS, FOODS TO AVOID, and SMART FOOD COMBINATIONS that promote ENERGY STABILITY and STRESS RESILIENCE.

CORTISOL-FRIENDLY FOODS: NUTRIENTS THAT NOURISH BALANCE

1. MAGNESIUM-RICH FOODS: CALMING THE NERVOUS SYSTEM

Magnesium is often referred to as the ANTI-STRESS MINERAL. It plays a central role in RELAXING MUSCLES, REGULATING BLOOD SUGAR, and SUPPORTING ADRENAL HEALTH. When magnesium levels drop, cortisol levels tend to RISE, leading to increased TENSION and ANXIETY.

Key magnesium-rich foods include:

- LEAFY GREENS: Spinach, kale, and Swiss chard provide a steady source of magnesium.
- NUTS AND SEEDS: Almonds, cashews, pumpkin seeds, and sunflower seeds are portable, nutrient-packed snacks.
- AVOCADOS: Rich in magnesium, potassium, and healthy fats, they help STABILIZE BLOOD SUGAR.
- DARK CHOCOLATE: An indulgence that delivers magnesium and antioxidants—but choose varieties with AT LEAST 70% CACAO and no added sugar.

Adding magnesium to meals can create a CALMING EFFECT that lowers cortisol spikes.

2. VITAMIN C: FIGHTING STRESS WITH ANTIOXIDANTS

Vitamin C is critical for ADRENAL GLAND FUNCTION and COLLAGEN PRODUCTION. It helps counteract OXIDATIVE STRESS, a condition that occurs when FREE RADICALS damage cells under chronic stress.

Top vitamin C sources include:

- CITRUS FRUITS: Oranges, lemons, and grapefruits deliver a quick antioxidant boost.
- BERRIES: Strawberries, blueberries, and raspberries are rich in POLYPHENOLS that fight inflammation.
- BELL PEPPERS: Particularly red and yellow varieties, they pack more vitamin C than most fruits.
- KIWI AND PAPAYA: Tropical options loaded with vitamin C and digestive enzymes for GUT HEALTH.

Incorporating vitamin C-rich foods can STRENGTHEN IMMUNITY and BUFFER THE ADRENAL GLANDS from overwork.

3. OMEGA-3 FATTY ACIDS: TAMING INFLAMMATION

Chronic stress triggers SYSTEMIC INFLAMMATION, which exacerbates cortisol dysregulation. Omega-3 fatty acids act as NATURAL ANTI-INFLAMMATORIES, helping to restore CELLULAR BALANCE.

Essential sources of omega-3s:

- FATTY FISH: Salmon, mackerel, sardines, and anchovies are RICH IN EPA AND DHA.
- CHIA SEEDS AND FLAXSEEDS: Plant-based omega-3s (ALA) for vegetarians.
- WALNUTS: A crunchy source of healthy fats and antioxidants.
- ALGAL OIL SUPPLEMENTS: Ideal for vegans seeking concentrated EPA and DHA.

Consuming omega-3s PROTECTS THE BRAIN, REDUCES ANXIETY, and supports HORMONAL HARMONY.

4. PROTEIN-RICH OPTIONS: FUELING ENERGY STABILITY

Protein is essential for REPAIRING TISSUES, BALANCING BLOOD SUGAR, and CURBING CORTISOL SPIKES. It also stabilizes energy by SLOWING DIGESTION and PROLONGING SATIETY.

Recommended protein sources:

- LEAN MEATS: Chicken, turkey, and grass-fed beef provide high-quality amino acids.
- EGGS: Packed with B VITAMINS and CHOLINE, they support NERVE HEALTH.
- LEGUMES: Lentils, chickpeas, and black beans deliver PLANT-BASED PROTEIN and FIBER.
- TOFU AND TEMPEH: Excellent vegetarian options rich in ISOFLAVONES that regulate hormones.

Balancing protein with FIBER and HEALTHY FATS prevents BLOOD SUGAR CRASHES that trigger cortisol release.

FOODS TO AVOID: CORTISOL TRIGGERS IN YOUR DIET

1. REFINED SUGAR: THE STRESS AMPLIFIER

Sugar causes RAPID BLOOD SUGAR SPIKES followed by crashes, forcing the adrenal glands to pump out MORE CORTISOL to stabilize energy. Chronic sugar intake fuels INFLAMMATION, INSULIN RESISTANCE, and MOOD SWINGS.

Hidden sources of sugar include:

- SODA AND SWEETENED BEVERAGES: Even so-called "healthy" drinks like SPORTS DRINKS or FRUIT JUICES.
- PASTRIES AND DESSERTS: Muffins, cakes, and cookies are REFINED CARB BOMBS.
- FLAVORED YOGURTS: Often marketed as healthy, they're loaded with added sugar.

2. CAFFEINE: OVERSTIMULATING THE ADRENALS

While caffeine provides a TEMPORARY ENERGY BOOST, it overstimulates the adrenal glands, keeping cortisol ELEVATED. High caffeine intake can also DISRUPT SLEEP CYCLES, creating a FEEDBACK LOOP of stress and fatigue.

Common sources to limit:

- COFFEE AND ESPRESSO: Swap for HERBAL TEAS or MATCHA, which offer GENTLER ENERGY.
- ENERGY DRINKS: Often overloaded with SUGAR and ARTIFICIAL STIMULANTS.
- DARK CHOCOLATE: While healthy in moderation, excess caffeine in cacao can be problematic.

3. PROCESSED FOODS: HIDDEN CHEMICALS AND ADDITIVES

Highly processed foods often contain PRESERVATIVES, ARTIFICIAL FLAVORS, and TRANS FATS that burden the DIGESTIVE SYSTEM and TRIGGER INFLAMMATION. Many also lack NUTRIENTS that support adrenal health.

Examples to watch out for:

- FROZEN MEALS: Loaded with SODIUM and PRESERVATIVES.
- CHIPS AND CRACKERS: Refined carbs that spike BLOOD SUGAR.
- FAST FOOD: Often fried in INFLAMMATORY OILS and lacking FIBER.

HOW TO COMBINE FOODS FOR STEADY ENERGY AND LOWER STRESS

1. BALANCING MACRONUTRIENTS

Pairing PROTEINS, HEALTHY FATS, and FIBER-RICH CARBS keeps BLOOD SUGAR STABLE and reduces the NEED FOR CORTISOL RELEASE. For example:

- BREAKFAST: Scrambled eggs with avocado and spinach.
- LUNCH: Quinoa salad with grilled salmon, olive oil, and roasted vegetables.
- DINNER: Roasted chicken, sweet potatoes, and steamed broccoli.

2. TIMING YOUR MEALS

Skipping meals or eating erratically sends signals of SCARCITY, triggering cortisol spikes. Instead:

- Eat REGULAR MEALS every 3–4 hours.
- Include PROTEIN-RICH SNACKS like almonds or hummus between meals.
- Avoid LATE-NIGHT EATING, which disrupts the CIRCADIAN RHYTHM.

3. PRIORITIZING ANTI-INFLAMMATORY INGREDIENTS

Spices and herbs such as TURMERIC, GINGER, and CINNAMON have CORTISOL-LOWERING PROPERTIES. Add them liberally to dishes and teas.

FINAL THOUGHTS ON FOOD AS MEDICINE

Food is more than sustenance—it's a TOOL for HORMONAL HEALING. By focusing on NUTRIENT-DENSE CHOICES and avoiding STRESS-TRIGGERING FOODS, you can REWIRE YOUR BODY'S STRESS RESPONSE. Small dietary changes create PROFOUND SHIFTS in how your body PRODUCES AND PROCESSES CORTISOL. The strategies in this section provide a FOUNDATION for VIBRANT ENERGY, CALM FOCUS, and LASTING WELLNESS.

3.2 RECIPES TO SUPPORT CORTISOL BALANCE

What we eat has the power to CALM THE NERVOUS SYSTEM, BALANCE HORMONES, and REDUCE INFLAMMATION. When building a cortisol-friendly diet, it's not just about avoiding harmful foods—it's about EMBRACING MEALS that nourish and RESTORE EQUILIBRIUM.

This section features recipes specifically designed to STABILIZE CORTISOL LEVELS, FUEL ENERGY, and SUPPORT RECOVERY. Each recipe emphasizes WHOLE FOODS, ANTI-INFLAMMATORY INGREDIENTS, and KEY NUTRIENTS like MAGNESIUM, VITAMIN C, and OMEGA-3 FATTY ACIDS.

Each recipe in this section is designed to serve **one portion**, making them quick and easy to prepare. You'll find **detailed instructions** and a **nutritional breakdown** highlighting the key benefits of each ingredient. These recipes are crafted to help you feel **grounded**, **focused**, and **energized** while supporting **hormonal balance** and **reducing inflammation**.

BREAKFASTS: STRESS-BUSTING STARTS TO YOUR DAY

1. MAGNESIUM-RICH OVERNIGHT OATS

Ingredients:
- ½ cup rolled oats
- 1 cup almond milk (unsweetened)
- 1 tablespoon chia seeds
- 1 small banana, sliced
- 1 tablespoon cacao nibs

Instructions:
1. Combine oats, almond milk, and chia seeds in a jar or bowl. Stir well.
2. Refrigerate overnight or for at least 4 hours until thickened.
3. Before serving, top with banana slices and cacao nibs.

Nutritional Benefits:
- ⇨ **MAGNESIUM:** Helps RELAX MUSCLES and REGULATE CORTISOL.
- ⇨ **FIBER:** Supports GUT HEALTH and SLOW ENERGY RELEASE.
- ⇨ **ANTIOXIDANTS:** Protect against OXIDATIVE STRESS.

2. ANTI-ANXIETY GREEN SMOOTHIE

Ingredients:

- 1 cup spinach
- ½ avocado
- 1 banana
- 1 tablespoon almond butter
- 1 cup coconut water
- 1 teaspoon spirulina powder

Instructions:
1. Blend all ingredients until smooth.
2. Add more coconut water if needed to reach the desired consistency.

Nutritional Benefits:
- ⇨ **B VITAMINS:** Vital for ADRENAL FUNCTION and ENERGY PRODUCTION.
- ⇨ **HEALTHY FATS:** Provide BRAIN-BOOSTING support and REDUCE INFLAMMATION.
- ⇨ **SPIRULINA:** A superfood rich in MINERALS to NOURISH ADRENALS.

3. PROTEIN-PACKED EGG MUFFINS

Ingredients (2 muffins):
- 2 large eggs
- ¼ cup spinach, chopped
- ¼ cup bell peppers, diced
- ¼ cup mushrooms, diced
- 2 tablespoons feta cheese
- Salt and pepper to taste

Instructions:
1. Preheat oven to 375°F (190°C). Grease a muffin tin.
2. Whisk eggs, salt, and pepper in a bowl.
3. Stir in vegetables and feta cheese.
4. Pour the mixture into muffin cups and bake for 18–20 minutes until set.

Nutritional Benefits:
- ⇨ **PROTEIN:** Supports MUSCLE REPAIR and HORMONE PRODUCTION.
- ⇨ **VEGETABLES:** Provide VITAMINS and MINERALS for STRESS RELIEF.
- ⇨ **FETA CHEESE:** Adds CALCIUM and PROBIOTICS for GUT HEALTH.

4. SWEET POTATO AND AVOCADO TOAST

Ingredients:
- 2 slices roasted sweet potato (½-inch thick)
- ½ avocado, smashed
- 1 teaspoon hemp seeds
- Pinch of sea salt and chili flakes

Instructions:
1. Roast sweet potato slices at 400°F (200°C) for 20 minutes or until tender.
2. Spread mashed avocado on each slice.
3. Sprinkle with hemp seeds, sea salt, and chili flakes.

Nutritional Benefits:
- ⇨ **COMPLEX CARBS:** Sustain ENERGY without SPIKES.
- ⇨ **HEALTHY FATS:** Stabilize HORMONES and CURB CRAVINGS.
- ⇨ **HEMP SEEDS:** Provide PLANT-BASED PROTEIN and OMEGA-3S.

5. GOLDEN TURMERIC LATTE

Ingredients:
- 1 cup almond milk
- ½ teaspoon turmeric powder
- ¼ teaspoon cinnamon
- Pinch of black pepper
- 1 teaspoon honey

Instructions:
1. Heat almond milk in a saucepan until warm.
2. Whisk in turmeric, cinnamon, black pepper, and honey until frothy.
3. Pour into a mug and enjoy warm.

Nutritional Benefits:
⇨ **TURMERIC:** Contains CURCUMIN, which fights INFLAMMATION.
⇨ **CINNAMON:** Balances BLOOD SUGAR LEVELS.
⇨ **BLACK PEPPER:** Enhances CURCUMIN ABSORPTION.

---

6. QUINOA BREAKFAST BOWL

Ingredients:
- ½ cup cooked quinoa
- ½ cup almond milk
- ¼ cup blueberries
- 1 tablespoon walnuts
- 1 teaspoon chia seeds

Instructions:
1. Combine quinoa and almond milk in a bowl.
2. Top with blueberries, walnuts, and chia seeds.

Nutritional Benefits:
⇨ **PROTEIN-RICH QUINOA:** Keeps CORTISOL STEADY.
⇨ **CHIA SEEDS:** Offer FIBER and OMEGA-3S.
⇨ **BLUEBERRIES:** Packed with ANTIOXIDANTS.

---

7. BANANA CHIA PUDDING

Ingredients:
- 3 tablespoons chia seeds
- 1 cup coconut milk
- 1 banana, mashed
- ½ teaspoon vanilla extract

Instructions:
1. Stir chia seeds, coconut milk, banana, and vanilla extract in a bowl.
2. Refrigerate overnight or for 4 hours until thick.

Nutritional Benefits:
⇨ **OMEGA-3S:** Reduce INFLAMMATION.
⇨ **FIBER:** Improves GUT HEALTH.
⇨ **BANANAS:** Provide POTASSIUM and CALM MUSCLES.

8. ALMOND BUTTER PROTEIN PANCAKES

Ingredients:
- ½ cup almond flour
- 1 egg
- 1 tablespoon almond butter
- ½ teaspoon vanilla extract

Instructions:
1. Mix all ingredients in a bowl until smooth.
2. Cook on a non-stick pan over medium heat until golden brown.

Nutritional Benefits:
- ⇨ **PROTEIN:** Builds MUSCLE and supports ADRENALS.
- ⇨ **HEALTHY FATS:** Provide LONG-LASTING ENERGY.
- ⇨ **ALMONDS:** Add MAGNESIUM to REDUCE STRESS.

---

9. COCONUT MATCHA SMOOTHIE

Ingredients:
- 1 cup coconut milk
- 1 teaspoon matcha powder
- ½ cup spinach
- ½ cup frozen mango
- 1 tablespoon flaxseeds

Instructions:
1. Blend all ingredients until smooth.

Nutritional Benefits:
- ⇨ **L-THEANINE:** Boosts FOCUS and REDUCES ANXIETY.
- ⇨ **FLAXSEEDS:** Provide OMEGA-3S and FIBER.
- ⇨ **MANGO:** Adds VITAMIN C to FIGHT OXIDATIVE STRESS.

---

10. ALMOND BUTTER AND BANANA SMOOTHIE

Ingredients:
- 1 banana
- 1 tablespoon almond butter
- 1 cup almond milk
- 1 handful spinach
- 1 tablespoon chia seeds

Instructions:
1. Combine all ingredients in a blender and blend until smooth.
2. Adjust consistency by adding more almond milk if needed.

Nutritional Benefits:
- ⇨ **BANANAS:** High in POTASSIUM to REDUCE MUSCLE TENSION.
- ⇨ **ALMOND BUTTER:** Provides HEALTHY FATS for HORMONAL BALANCE.
- ⇨ **CHIA SEEDS:** Boost OMEGA-3S and FIBER for GUT HEALTH.

11. GREEK YOGURT PARFAIT WITH BERRIES AND GRANOLA

Ingredients:
- ¾ cup Greek yogurt (unsweetened)
- ½ cup mixed berries (blueberries, raspberries, strawberries)
- 2 tablespoons granola
- 1 teaspoon flaxseeds

Instructions:
1. Layer Greek yogurt, berries, and granola in a glass or bowl.
2. Sprinkle flaxseeds on top and enjoy immediately.

Nutritional Benefits:
- ⇨ **PROBIOTICS:** Support GUT HEALTH, which directly impacts STRESS RESILIENCE.
- ⇨ **ANTIOXIDANTS:** Combat OXIDATIVE STRESS.
- ⇨ **GRANOLA:** Adds FIBER for STEADY DIGESTION.

---

12. SWEET POTATO AND EGG BREAKFAST BOWL

Ingredients:
- 1 small roasted sweet potato, cubed
- 2 scrambled eggs
- ½ avocado, sliced
- 1 handful spinach, sautéed
- Salt and pepper to taste

Instructions:
1. Roast sweet potato cubes at 400°F (200°C) for 20 minutes or until tender.
2. Scramble eggs in a non-stick pan.
3. Assemble the bowl with sweet potatoes, eggs, avocado, and sautéed spinach.
4. Season with salt and pepper.

Nutritional Benefits:
- ⇨ **SWEET POTATO:** Provides COMPLEX CARBS for SUSTAINED ENERGY.
- ⇨ **EGGS:** Deliver PROTEIN to SUPPORT ADRENAL FUNCTION.
- ⇨ **AVOCADO:** Offers HEALTHY FATS and FIBER.

---

13. CHIA SEED PUDDING WITH ALMOND MILK AND BERRIES

Ingredients:
- 3 tablespoons chia seeds
- 1 cup almond milk (unsweetened)
- ½ teaspoon vanilla extract
- ½ cup mixed berries

Instructions:
1. Combine chia seeds, almond milk, and vanilla extract in a jar or bowl. Stir well.
2. Refrigerate overnight or at least 4 hours until thickened.
3. Top with berries before serving.

Nutritional Benefits:
- ⇨ **OMEGA-3 FATTY ACIDS:** Combat INFLAMMATION and SUPPORT CORTISOL BALANCE.
- ⇨ **FIBER:** Keeps DIGESTION SMOOTH and ENERGY LEVELS STABLE.
- ⇨ **ANTIOXIDANTS:** Protect against STRESS-INDUCED DAMAGE.

14. BLUEBERRY ALMOND SMOOTHIE BOWL

Ingredients:
- 1 cup frozen blueberries
- 1 banana
- ½ cup almond milk
- 1 tablespoon almond butter
- 1 tablespoon chia seeds
- 2 tablespoons granola (optional topping)

Instructions:
1. Blend blueberries, banana, almond milk, almond butter, and chia seeds until smooth.
2. Pour into a bowl and top with granola if desired.

Nutritional Benefits:
- ⇨ **BLUEBERRIES:** High in ANTIOXIDANTS to COMBAT FREE RADICALS.
- ⇨ **CHIA SEEDS:** Provide FIBER and OMEGA-3S.
- ⇨ **ALMOND BUTTER:** Adds HEALTHY FATS for HORMONAL SUPPORT.

---

15. PUMPKIN SPICE SMOOTHIE

Ingredients:
- ½ cup pumpkin puree
- 1 frozen banana
- 1 cup almond milk
- 1 teaspoon pumpkin pie spice
- 1 tablespoon flaxseeds
- 1 teaspoon maple syrup

Instructions:
1. Blend all ingredients until smooth.
2. Adjust sweetness with maple syrup, if needed.

Nutritional Benefits:
- ⇨ **PUMPKIN:** High in VITAMIN A and FIBER.
- ⇨ **FLAXSEEDS:** Offer OMEGA-3S and ANTI-INFLAMMATORY BENEFITS.
- ⇨ **BANANA:** Provides NATURAL SUGARS for a GENTLE ENERGY BOOST.

---

16. APPLE CINNAMON QUINOA PORRIDGE

Ingredients:
- ½ cup cooked quinoa
- ½ cup almond milk
- ½ apple, diced
- ½ teaspoon cinnamon
- 1 teaspoon honey

Instructions:
1. Warm cooked quinoa and almond milk in a saucepan.
2. Stir in diced apple and cinnamon.
3. Drizzle honey on top before serving.

Nutritional Benefits:
- ⇨ **QUINOA:** A COMPLETE PROTEIN for ENERGY BALANCE.
- ⇨ **CINNAMON:** Stabilizes BLOOD SUGAR LEVELS.
- ⇨ **APPLES:** Provide FIBER and NATURAL SWEETNESS.

LUNCHES: ANTI-INFLAMMATORY AND SATISFYING MEALS

1. GRILLED SALMON QUINOA BOWL

Ingredients:
- 1 grilled salmon fillet (about 4 oz)
- ½ cup cooked quinoa
- 1 cup chopped kale (massaged with olive oil)
- ½ avocado, sliced
- 2 tablespoons lemon-tahini dressing

Instructions:
1. Cook quinoa according to package instructions.
2. Grill the salmon until fully cooked, about 4–5 minutes per side.
3. Massage kale with a drizzle of olive oil to soften.
4. Assemble the bowl by layering quinoa, kale, and avocado slices.
5. Top with grilled salmon and drizzle with lemon-tahini dressing.

Nutritional Benefits:
- ⇨ **SALMON:** Rich in OMEGA-3 FATTY ACIDS to REDUCE INFLAMMATION.
- ⇨ **QUINOA:** Provides PLANT-BASED PROTEIN and FIBER for GUT HEALTH.
- ⇨ **KALE:** Packed with ANTIOXIDANTS to SUPPORT DETOXIFICATION.

---

2. MEDITERRANEAN CHICKPEA SALAD

Ingredients:
- ½ cup canned chickpeas (rinsed and drained)
- ½ cucumber, diced
- ½ cup cherry tomatoes, halved
- 2 tablespoons sliced olives
- ¼ red onion, thinly sliced
- 1 tablespoon olive oil
- 1 teaspoon lemon juice
- 1 tablespoon crumbled feta cheese (optional)

Instructions:
1. Combine chickpeas, cucumber, tomatoes, olives, and red onion in a bowl.
2. Drizzle with olive oil and lemon juice. Toss well.
3. Top with feta cheese, if desired.

Nutritional Benefits:
- ⇨ **CHICKPEAS:** High in FIBER and PLANT-BASED PROTEIN to STABILIZE BLOOD SUGAR.
- ⇨ **OLIVE OIL:** Provides HEALTHY FATS to REDUCE INFLAMMATION.
- ⇨ **TOMATOES:** Rich in VITAMIN C and LYCOPENE for ANTIOXIDANT PROTECTION.

3. TURKEY AND SWEET POTATO WRAPS

Ingredients:
- 2 slices roasted turkey breast (nitrate-free)
- ½ cup roasted sweet potato slices
- ½ cup arugula
- 2 tablespoons hummus
- 1 whole-grain tortilla

Instructions:
1. Spread hummus on the tortilla.
2. Layer with turkey slices, roasted sweet potatoes, and arugula.
3. Roll the tortilla tightly and slice in half.

Nutritional Benefits:
- ⇨ **TURKEY:** Provides LEAN PROTEIN to SUPPORT MUSCLE RECOVERY.
- ⇨ **SWEET POTATO:** Rich in COMPLEX CARBS and VITAMIN A for ENERGY.
- ⇨ **HUMMUS:** Adds FIBER and HEALTHY FATS for SUSTAINED ENERGY.

4. LENTIL DETOX SOUP

Ingredients:
- ½ cup green lentils
- 1 carrot, diced
- 1 celery stalk, diced
- 1 handful spinach
- ½ teaspoon turmeric
- 2 cups vegetable broth

Instructions:
1. Rinse lentils and add them to a pot with vegetable broth. Bring to a boil.
2. Add carrots, celery, and turmeric. Simmer for 20–25 minutes until lentils are tender.
3. Stir in spinach and let it wilt. Serve warm.

Nutritional Benefits:
- ⇨ **LENTILS:** High in FIBER and PLANT PROTEIN for DIGESTIVE HEALTH.
- ⇨ **TURMERIC:** Contains CURCUMIN to REDUCE INFLAMMATION.
- ⇨ **SPINACH:** Provides MAGNESIUM and IRON for ENERGY PRODUCTION.

5. TUNA AND AVOCADO LETTUCE WRAPS

Ingredients:
- 1 can tuna (packed in water), drained
- ½ avocado, mashed
- 1 tablespoon Greek yogurt
- 1 teaspoon lemon juice
- 3 romaine lettuce leaves

Instructions:
1. Mix tuna, mashed avocado, Greek yogurt, and lemon juice.
2. Spoon the mixture into romaine leaves and serve.

Nutritional Benefits:
- ⇨ **TUNA:** High in OMEGA-3S to REDUCE INFLAMMATION.
- ⇨ **AVOCADO:** Provides FIBER and HEALTHY FATS for BRAIN SUPPORT.
- ⇨ **GREEK YOGURT:** Adds PROBIOTICS for GUT HEALTH.

6. QUINOA AND ROASTED VEGGIE BOWL

Ingredients:
- ½ cup cooked quinoa
- ½ cup roasted zucchini slices
- ½ cup roasted carrots
- ½ cup roasted beets
- 1 tablespoon tahini drizzle

Instructions:
1. Roast vegetables at 400°F for 20 minutes, tossing halfway.
2. Cook quinoa as directed.
3. Assemble the bowl with quinoa and roasted veggies.
4. Drizzle with tahini before serving.

Nutritional Benefits:
- ⇨ **QUINOA:** Provides COMPLETE PROTEIN and FIBER.
- ⇨ **BEETS:** Boost ANTIOXIDANTS and DETOXIFICATION.
- ⇨ **TAHINI:** Adds CALCIUM and HEALTHY FATS to BALANCE HORMONES.

---

7. ASIAN CHICKEN SALAD

Ingredients:
- 1 grilled chicken breast (4 oz), sliced
- 1 cup shredded cabbage
- ½ cup shredded carrots
- 1 teaspoon sesame oil
- 1 tablespoon ginger dressing

Instructions:
1. Toss cabbage and carrots in sesame oil and ginger dressing.
2. Top with grilled chicken slices.

Nutritional Benefits:
- ⇨ **CHICKEN:** Provides LEAN PROTEIN for MUSCLE REPAIR.
- ⇨ **GINGER:** Offers ANTI-INFLAMMATORY benefits.
- ⇨ **CABBAGE:** Supports DIGESTION and DETOXIFICATION.

---

8. SPICY LENTIL AND KALE BOWL

Ingredients:
- ½ cup cooked lentils
- 1 cup chopped kale (massaged with olive oil)
- ½ cup roasted sweet potatoes
- ¼ teaspoon chili flakes

Instructions:
1. Cook lentils as directed.
2. Massage kale with olive oil to soften.
3. Assemble the bowl with lentils, kale, and roasted sweet potatoes.
4. Sprinkle with chili flakes for heat.

Nutritional Benefits:
- ⇨ **LENTILS:** Provide PLANT PROTEIN and IRON for ENERGY.
- ⇨ **KALE:** Boosts MAGNESIUM for STRESS RELIEF.
- ⇨ **SWEET POTATOES:** Offer COMPLEX CARBS for SUSTAINED ENERGY.

9. AVOCADO AND SHRIMP SALAD

Ingredients:
- 4 oz cooked shrimp (peeled and deveined)
- ½ avocado, diced
- 1 cup arugula
- ½ cucumber, sliced
- 1 tablespoon lime juice
- 1 teaspoon olive oil
- Salt and pepper to taste

Instructions:
1. Toss arugula, avocado, cucumber, and shrimp in a bowl.
2. Drizzle with lime juice and olive oil.
3. Season with salt and pepper.

Nutritional Benefits:
- ⇨ **SHRIMP:** High in PROTEIN and SELENIUM for IMMUNE SUPPORT.
- ⇨ **AVOCADO:** Provides HEALTHY FATS and FIBER for HORMONE BALANCE.
- ⇨ **ARUGULA:** Rich in ANTIOXIDANTS and VITAMINS to REDUCE INFLAMMATION.

---

10. TURKEY ZUCCHINI BOATS

Ingredients:
- 1 medium zucchini, halved lengthwise and hollowed out
- 4 oz ground turkey
- ¼ cup marinara sauce
- 2 tablespoons grated Parmesan cheese
- 1 teaspoon olive oil
- Salt and pepper to taste

Instructions:
1. Preheat oven to 375°F.
2. Sauté ground turkey in olive oil until cooked. Add marinara sauce and mix well.
3. Stuff the zucchini halves with the turkey mixture.
4. Sprinkle with Parmesan cheese.
5. Bake for 20 minutes or until zucchini is tender.

Nutritional Benefits:
- ⇨ **TURKEY:** Lean PROTEIN for MUSCLE RECOVERY.
- ⇨ **ZUCCHINI:** Low in CARBS and rich in VITAMINS for DIGESTIVE HEALTH.
- ⇨ **PARMESAN:** Provides CALCIUM and UMAMI FLAVOR.

11. GRILLED TURKEY AND AVOCADO WRAP

Ingredients:
- 1 whole-grain tortilla
- 3 oz roasted turkey breast
- ½ avocado, sliced
- ½ cup baby spinach
- 1 tablespoon hummus

Instructions:
1. Spread hummus on the tortilla.
2. Layer turkey, avocado, and spinach.
3. Roll tightly and slice in half.

Nutritional Benefits:
- ⇨ **TURKEY:** Provides LEAN PROTEIN to REDUCE INFLAMMATION.
- ⇨ **AVOCADO:** Supports HORMONAL HEALTH with HEALTHY FATS.
- ⇨ **SPINACH:** Rich in MAGNESIUM for STRESS RELIEF.

---

12. LENTIL AND SWEET POTATO BUDDHA BOWL

Ingredients:
- ½ cup cooked lentils
- ½ cup roasted sweet potatoes
- 1 cup kale, massaged with olive oil
- 1 tablespoon tahini dressing
- 1 tablespoon pumpkin seeds

Instructions:
1. Cook lentils as directed.
2. Roast sweet potatoes at 400°F for 20 minutes until soft.
3. Massage kale with olive oil to soften.
4. Assemble all ingredients in a bowl and drizzle with tahini dressing.
5. Top with pumpkin seeds.

Nutritional Benefits:
- ⇨ **LENTILS:** Provide FIBER and IRON for ENERGY PRODUCTION.
- ⇨ **SWEET POTATOES:** Packed with VITAMIN A and COMPLEX CARBS.
- ⇨ **PUMPKIN SEEDS:** Rich in MAGNESIUM and ZINC to SUPPORT ADRENAL HEALTH.

13. GRILLED CHICKEN AND AVOCADO SALAD

Ingredients:
- 4 oz grilled chicken breast
- 2 cups mixed greens
- ½ avocado, sliced
- ½ cup cherry tomatoes, halved
- 1 tablespoon sunflower seeds
- 1 tablespoon balsamic vinaigrette

Instructions:
1. Toss greens, tomatoes, and sunflower seeds in a bowl.
2. Top with grilled chicken and avocado slices.
3. Drizzle with balsamic vinaigrette.

Nutritional Benefits:
- ⇨ **CHICKEN:** Lean PROTEIN to SUPPORT MUSCLE REPAIR.
- ⇨ **AVOCADO:** Provides HEALTHY FATS for HORMONAL BALANCE.
- ⇨ **SUNFLOWER SEEDS:** High in VITAMIN E and MAGNESIUM for STRESS RELIEF.

---

14. THAI QUINOA AND EDAMAME SALAD

Ingredients:
- ½ cup cooked quinoa
- ½ cup shelled edamame
- ¼ cup shredded carrots
- ¼ cup shredded purple cabbage
- 1 teaspoon sesame seeds
- 1 tablespoon peanut-ginger dressing

Instructions:
1. Cook quinoa and let it cool.
2. Toss with edamame, carrots, and cabbage.
3. Drizzle with peanut-ginger dressing and sprinkle sesame seeds on top.

Nutritional Benefits:
- ⇨ **QUINOA:** Provides COMPLETE PROTEIN and FIBER.
- ⇨ **EDAMAME:** Rich in PLANT-BASED PROTEIN and ANTIOXIDANTS.
- ⇨ **GINGER:** Supports DIGESTION and ANTI-INFLAMMATORY RESPONSES.

15. SALMON AND BROWN RICE BOWL WITH AVOCADO DRESSING

Ingredients:
- ½ cup cooked brown rice
- 4 oz grilled salmon
- ½ cup steamed broccoli
- 1 tablespoon avocado dressing
- 1 teaspoon sesame seeds

Instructions:
1. Cook brown rice and steam broccoli.
2. Grill salmon until cooked through.
3. Assemble rice, salmon, and broccoli in a bowl.
4. Drizzle with avocado dressing and sprinkle sesame seeds.

Nutritional Benefits:
- ⇨ **SALMON:** High in OMEGA-3S for BRAIN HEALTH.
- ⇨ **BROWN RICE:** Provides COMPLEX CARBS and FIBER for ENERGY.
- ⇨ **BROCCOLI:** Packed with VITAMINS C AND K to REDUCE INFLAMMATION.

---

16. STUFFED BELL PEPPERS WITH TURKEY AND SPINACH

Ingredients:
- 1 large bell pepper, halved and hollowed
- 4 oz ground turkey
- ½ cup cooked brown rice
- ½ cup chopped spinach
- 2 tablespoons marinara sauce
- 1 tablespoon Parmesan cheese

Instructions:
1. Preheat oven to 375°F.
2. Cook turkey in a skillet until browned. Add spinach and stir until wilted.
3. Mix in cooked rice and marinara sauce.
4. Stuff bell pepper halves with the mixture.
5. Sprinkle Parmesan cheese on top. Bake for 20 minutes.

Nutritional Benefits:
- ⇨ **TURKEY:** Lean PROTEIN to SUPPORT METABOLISM.
- ⇨ **SPINACH:** High in IRON and MAGNESIUM for STRESS RECOVERY.
- ⇨ **BELL PEPPERS:** Rich in VITAMIN C and ANTIOXIDANTS.

DINNERS: RESTORATIVE AND HEALING MEALS

1. MISO DETOX SOUP

Ingredients:
- 1 tablespoon miso paste
- 1 cup water
- ¼ cup seaweed (wakame or nori), rehydrated
- ¼ cup sliced mushrooms (shiitake or button)
- 2 oz tofu, cubed
- 1 green onion, sliced

Instructions:
1. Bring water to a simmer in a small pot.
2. Add mushrooms and cook for 3–4 minutes until softened.
3. Stir in tofu and seaweed. Simmer for 2 minutes.
4. Remove from heat and dissolve miso paste in a small bowl with some hot broth.
5. Stir miso mixture back into the pot.
6. Garnish with green onions and serve warm.

Nutritional Benefits:
- ⇨ **MISO:** Provides PROBIOTICS for GUT HEALTH.
- ⇨ **SEAWEED:** High in IODINE and MINERALS to SUPPORT THYROID FUNCTION.
- ⇨ **TOFU:** Offers PLANT-BASED PROTEIN and CALCIUM.

---

2. LEMON HERB BAKED COD

Ingredients:
- 1 cod fillet (5–6 oz)
- 1 garlic clove, minced
- 1 tablespoon lemon juice
- 1 teaspoon olive oil
- 1 teaspoon fresh herbs (parsley, dill, or thyme)
- Salt and pepper to taste

Instructions:
1. Preheat oven to 400°F.
2. Place cod fillet on a baking sheet lined with parchment paper.
3. Drizzle with olive oil and lemon juice.
4. Sprinkle with garlic, herbs, salt, and pepper.
5. Bake for 12–15 minutes until fish flakes easily.

Nutritional Benefits:
- ⇨ **COD:** High in LEAN PROTEIN and OMEGA-3S to REDUCE INFLAMMATION.
- ⇨ **LEMON:** Rich in VITAMIN C to SUPPORT IMMUNITY.
- ⇨ **OLIVE OIL:** Provides HEALTHY FATS for HEART HEALTH.

3. TURMERIC CHICKEN CURRY

Ingredients:
- 4 oz chicken breast, diced
- ½ cup coconut milk
- 1 cup spinach
- 1 garlic clove, minced
- ½ teaspoon turmeric
- ½ teaspoon cumin
- 1 teaspoon olive oil

Instructions:
1. Heat olive oil in a skillet over medium heat.
2. Sauté garlic until fragrant, about 1 minute.
3. Add chicken and cook until browned.
4. Stir in turmeric and cumin.
5. Pour in coconut milk and simmer for 10 minutes.
6. Add spinach and cook until wilted.

Nutritional Benefits:
- ⇨ **CHICKEN:** Lean PROTEIN for MUSCLE REPAIR.
- ⇨ **TURMERIC:** Powerful ANTI-INFLAMMATORY properties.
- ⇨ **COCONUT MILK:** Provides HEALTHY FATS to STABILIZE BLOOD SUGAR.

---

4. STUFFED BELL PEPPERS

Ingredients:
- 1 large bell pepper, halved and deseeded
- 4 oz ground turkey
- ¼ cup cooked brown rice
- 2 tablespoons diced tomatoes
- 2 tablespoons black beans

Instructions:
1. Preheat oven to 375°F.
2. Cook ground turkey in a skillet until browned.
3. Mix turkey with rice, tomatoes, and black beans.
4. Stuff mixture into bell pepper halves.
5. Bake for 20 minutes.

Nutritional Benefits:
- ⇨ **TURKEY:** Provides LEAN PROTEIN for MUSCLE RECOVERY.
- ⇨ **BLACK BEANS:** High in FIBER to SUPPORT DIGESTION.
- ⇨ **BELL PEPPERS:** Rich in VITAMIN C and ANTIOXIDANTS.

5. WILD RICE AND VEGGIE STIR-FRY

Ingredients:
- ½ cup cooked wild rice
- ½ cup broccoli florets
- ½ cup sliced carrots
- 1 teaspoon sesame oil
- ½ teaspoon grated ginger

Instructions:
1. Heat sesame oil in a skillet over medium heat.
2. Sauté carrots and broccoli until tender, about 5 minutes.
3. Stir in cooked wild rice and ginger.
4. Cook for 2–3 minutes until heated through.

Nutritional Benefits:
- ⇨ **WILD RICE:** Provides FIBER and COMPLEX CARBS for ENERGY BALANCE.
- ⇨ **BROCCOLI:** High in VITAMINS C AND K to REDUCE INFLAMMATION.
- ⇨ **SESAME OIL:** Adds HEALTHY FATS for HORMONAL SUPPORT.

---

6. SALMON AND ASPARAGUS FOIL PACKETS

Ingredients:
- 1 salmon fillet (5–6 oz)
- 6 asparagus spears
- 1 tablespoon olive oil
- 2 lemon slices
- Salt and pepper to taste

Instructions:
1. Preheat oven to 400°F.
2. Place salmon and asparagus on a piece of foil.
3. Drizzle with olive oil and season with salt and pepper.
4. Top with lemon slices.
5. Seal foil packet and bake for 15–20 minutes.

Nutritional Benefits:
- ⇨ **SALMON:** Rich in OMEGA-3 FATTY ACIDS for BRAIN HEALTH.
- ⇨ **ASPARAGUS:** Provides ANTIOXIDANTS and supports DETOXIFICATION.
- ⇨ **OLIVE OIL:** Adds ANTI-INFLAMMATORY FATS.

7. ROASTED CAULIFLOWER STEAKS

Ingredients:
- 1 large cauliflower slice (1-inch thick)
- 1 tablespoon tahini
- 1 garlic clove, minced
- ½ teaspoon paprika
- 1 teaspoon olive oil

Instructions:
1. Preheat oven to 400°F.
2. Brush cauliflower slice with olive oil and season with garlic and paprika.
3. Roast for 25–30 minutes until golden brown.
4. Drizzle with tahini before serving.

Nutritional Benefits:
- ⇨ **CAULIFLOWER:** Provides FIBER and ANTIOXIDANTS.
- ⇨ **TAHINI:** High in HEALTHY FATS and CALCIUM.
- ⇨ **GARLIC:** Offers ANTI-INFLAMMATORY and IMMUNE-BOOSTING properties.

---

8. BAKED CHICKEN AND QUINOA PILAF

Ingredients:
- 4 oz chicken breast
- ½ cup cooked quinoa
- ½ cup spinach
- 1 tablespoon slivered almonds

Instructions:
1. Preheat oven to 375°F.
2. Season chicken with salt and pepper and bake for 20–25 minutes.
3. Mix cooked quinoa with spinach and almonds.
4. Slice chicken and serve on top.

Nutritional Benefits:
- ⇨ **CHICKEN:** High in LEAN PROTEIN to REPAIR MUSCLES.
- ⇨ **QUINOA:** Provides FIBER and MAGNESIUM.
- ⇨ **ALMONDS:** Rich in VITAMIN E and HEALTHY FATS.

9. COCONUT CURRY LENTILS

Ingredients:
- ½ cup cooked lentils
- ½ cup coconut milk
- 1 garlic clove, minced
- ½ teaspoon grated ginger
- ½ teaspoon turmeric
- 1 cup spinach

Instructions:
1. Heat a saucepan over medium heat.
2. Sauté garlic and ginger until fragrant.
3. Add lentils, coconut milk, and turmeric. Simmer for 5 minutes.
4. Stir in spinach until wilted.

Nutritional Benefits:
- ⇨ LENTILS: High in FIBER and PLANT PROTEIN for DIGESTION AND SATIETY.
- ⇨ COCONUT MILK: Provides HEALTHY FATS to BALANCE HORMONES.
- ⇨ TURMERIC: Anti-inflammatory and supports IMMUNE HEALTH.

---

10. ZOODLE SHRIMP STIR-FRY

Ingredients:
- 1 cup zucchini noodles (zoodles)
- 4 oz shrimp, peeled and deveined
- 1 garlic clove, minced
- 1 teaspoon sesame oil
- 1 teaspoon coconut aminos or low-sodium soy sauce

Instructions:
1. Heat sesame oil in a skillet over medium heat.
2. Sauté garlic until fragrant, about 1 minute.
3. Add shrimp and cook until pink, about 3 minutes per side.
4. Stir in zoodles and coconut aminos. Cook for 2–3 minutes until tender.

Nutritional Benefits:
- ⇨ SHRIMP: High in LEAN PROTEIN and SELENIUM for METABOLISM SUPPORT.
- ⇨ ZOODLES: Low-carb and rich in VITAMINS A AND C.
- ⇨ SESAME OIL: Provides ANTI-INFLAMMATORY FATS.

11. BAKED LEMON HERB CHICKEN THIGHS

Ingredients:
- 2 bone-in chicken thighs
- 1 tablespoon olive oil
- 1 tablespoon lemon juice
- 1 garlic clove, minced
- ½ teaspoon dried thyme
- Salt and pepper to taste

Instructions:
1. Preheat oven to 400°F.
2. Mix olive oil, lemon juice, garlic, thyme, salt, and pepper.
3. Rub mixture onto chicken thighs.
4. Bake for 25–30 minutes until skin is golden and crispy.

Nutritional Benefits:
- ⇨ **CHICKEN THIGHS:** Rich in PROTEIN and COLLAGEN for MUSCLE REPAIR.
- ⇨ **LEMON:** Boosts VITAMIN C for IMMUNITY.
- ⇨ **OLIVE OIL:** Contains MONOUNSATURATED FATS for HEART HEALTH.

---

12. TURMERIC CAULIFLOWER RICE WITH GRILLED SHRIMP

Ingredients:
- 1 cup cauliflower rice
- 4 oz shrimp, peeled and deveined
- ½ teaspoon turmeric
- 1 teaspoon coconut oil
- 1 tablespoon chopped cilantro

Instructions:
1. Heat coconut oil in a skillet over medium heat.
2. Sauté shrimp until pink, about 3 minutes per side. Remove from skillet.
3. Add cauliflower rice and turmeric, cooking for 5 minutes until tender.
4. Stir in cilantro and top with grilled shrimp.

Nutritional Benefits:
- ⇨ **CAULIFLOWER RICE:** Low-carb and rich in FIBER.
- ⇨ **TURMERIC:** Provides ANTI-INFLAMMATORY benefits.
- ⇨ **SHRIMP:** High in PROTEIN and OMEGA-3 FATTY ACIDS.

13. LENTIL AND VEGETABLE CURRY

Ingredients:
- ½ cup red lentils, rinsed
- 1 cup coconut milk
- ½ cup spinach
- ½ cup diced carrots
- ½ teaspoon turmeric
- ¼ teaspoon cumin

Instructions:
1. In a saucepan, combine lentils, coconut milk, carrots, turmeric, and cumin.
2. Simmer for 15–20 minutes until lentils are soft.
3. Stir in spinach and cook until wilted.

Nutritional Benefits:
- ⇨ **LENTILS:** Provide FIBER and IRON for ENERGY PRODUCTION.
- ⇨ **COCONUT MILK:** Contains HEALTHY FATS to BALANCE HORMONES.
- ⇨ **TURMERIC:** Anti-inflammatory properties to REDUCE INFLAMMATION.

---

14. MUSHROOM AND SPINACH STIR-FRY

Ingredients:
- 1 cup sliced shiitake mushrooms
- 1 cup fresh spinach
- 1 garlic clove, minced
- 1 teaspoon sesame oil
- 1 teaspoon tamari (or soy sauce)

Instructions:
1. Heat sesame oil in a skillet over medium heat.
2. Sauté garlic until fragrant.
3. Add mushrooms and cook for 5 minutes until softened.
4. Stir in spinach and tamari. Cook until wilted.

Nutritional Benefits:
- ⇨ **MUSHROOMS:** High in SELENIUM and ANTIOXIDANTS for IMMUNE HEALTH.
- ⇨ **SPINACH:** Provides IRON and MAGNESIUM.
- ⇨ **SESAME OIL:** Rich in ANTI-INFLAMMATORY FATS.

15. ROASTED VEGETABLE AND QUINOA BOWL

Ingredients:
- ½ cup cooked quinoa
- ½ cup roasted zucchini
- ½ cup roasted sweet potatoes
- ½ cup roasted bell peppers
- 1 tablespoon tahini sauce

Instructions:
1. Roast vegetables at 400°F for 20–25 minutes until tender.
2. Combine cooked quinoa and roasted vegetables in a bowl.
3. Drizzle with tahini sauce before serving.

Nutritional Benefits:
- ⇨ **QUINOA:** Provides FIBER and MAGNESIUM for ENERGY.
- ⇨ **VEGETABLES:** High in ANTIOXIDANTS to REDUCE INFLAMMATION.
- ⇨ **TAHINI:** Contains HEALTHY FATS and CALCIUM.

---

16. BEEF AND BROCCOLI STIR-FRY

Ingredients:
- 4 oz grass-fed beef, thinly sliced
- 1 cup broccoli florets
- 1 teaspoon grated ginger
- 1 garlic clove, minced
- 1 tablespoon coconut aminos (or low-sodium soy sauce)
- 1 teaspoon sesame oil

Instructions:
1. Heat sesame oil in a skillet over medium-high heat.
2. Add ginger and garlic, sauté until fragrant.
3. Add beef and stir-fry for 3–4 minutes until browned.
4. Toss in broccoli and coconut aminos, cooking for another 3 minutes until tender.

Nutritional Benefits:
- ⇨ **GRASS-FED BEEF:** High in IRON and ZINC for HORMONAL BALANCE.
- ⇨ **BROCCOLI:** Provides VITAMIN C and FIBER to SUPPORT DIGESTION.
- ⇨ **SESAME OIL:** Anti-inflammatory and rich in HEALTHY FATS.

17. LEMON HERB BAKED COD

Ingredients:
- 1 cod fillet (4–5 oz)
- 1 tablespoon lemon juice
- 1 garlic clove, minced
- 1 teaspoon olive oil
- 1 teaspoon fresh parsley, chopped
- Salt and pepper to taste

Instructions:
1. Preheat oven to 375°F.
2. Season cod with salt, pepper, lemon juice, garlic, and olive oil.
3. Bake for 12–15 minutes until fish flakes easily with a fork.
4. Garnish with parsley before serving.

Nutritional Benefits:
- ⇨ **COD:** High in PROTEIN and OMEGA-3 FATTY ACIDS for INFLAMMATION REDUCTION.
- ⇨ **LEMON:** Provides VITAMIN C to BOOST IMMUNITY.
- ⇨ **OLIVE OIL:** Contains MONOUNSATURATED FATS for HEART HEALTH.

---

18. CHICKEN ZOODLE SOUP

Ingredients:
- 1 cup zucchini noodles (zoodles)
- ½ cup shredded chicken breast
- ½ cup carrots, diced
- ½ cup celery, diced
- 1 cup bone broth
- Salt and pepper to taste

Instructions:
1. Heat bone broth in a pot over medium heat.
2. Add carrots and celery, simmer for 10 minutes until tender.
3. Stir in chicken and zoodles, cooking for 3–4 minutes until warmed through.
4. Season with salt and pepper before serving.

Nutritional Benefits:
- ⇨ **CHICKEN:** Lean PROTEIN for MUSCLE RECOVERY.
- ⇨ **ZOODLES:** Low-carb and rich in VITAMINS A AND C.
- ⇨ **BONE BROTH:** Supports GUT HEALTH and COLLAGEN PRODUCTION.

SNACKS: QUICK BOOSTS FOR ENERGY AND CALM

1. SPIRULINA ENERGY BALLS

Ingredients (3 balls):
- 5 Medjool dates, pitted
- 1 tbsp almond butter
- 1 tsp spirulina powder
- 1 tbsp chia seeds
- 1 tbsp cacao nibs

Instructions:
1. In a food processor, blend dates and almond butter until a smooth paste forms.
2. Add spirulina powder and chia seeds, then pulse until well combined.
3. Stir in cacao nibs.
4. Roll the mixture into 3 small balls and refrigerate for 15–20 minutes before serving.

Nutritional Benefits:
- ⇨ **SPIRULINA:** Rich in minerals like IRON and MAGNESIUM, promoting ENERGY PRODUCTION.
- ⇨ **CHIA SEEDS:** Provide OMEGA-3 FATTY ACIDS and FIBER for DIGESTIVE HEALTH.
- ⇨ **CACAO NIBS:** Packed with ANTIOXIDANTS and support MOOD ENHANCEMENT.

---

2. NUT AND SEED TRAIL MIX

Ingredients:
- 2 tbsp almonds
- 2 tbsp walnuts
- 1 tbsp pumpkin seeds
- 1 tbsp sunflower seeds
- 1 tbsp dried berries (e.g., goji berries or cranberries)

Instructions:
1. Mix all the ingredients in a small bowl or airtight container.
2. Store in a jar or bag for an on-the-go snack.

Nutritional Benefits:
- ⇨ **NUTS AND SEEDS:** Rich in MAGNESIUM, supporting STRESS RELIEF and MUSCLE RELAXATION.
- ⇨ **DRIED BERRIES:** Add ANTIOXIDANTS to fight OXIDATIVE STRESS.
- ⇨ Balanced combination of PROTEIN, FATS, and FIBER helps maintain steady ENERGY LEVELS.

---

3. AVOCADO AND SEA SALT RICE CAKES

Ingredients:
- 2 brown rice cakes
- 1/2 ripe avocado, sliced
- A pinch of sea salt

Instructions:
1. Top each rice cake with sliced avocado.
2. Sprinkle lightly with sea salt.

Nutritional Benefits:
- ⇨ **AVOCADO:** Provides HEALTHY FATS and POTASSIUM to support HYDRATION and ENERGY BALANCE.
- ⇨ **RICE CAKES:** Offer a GLUTEN-FREE CARB SOURCE to stabilize BLOOD SUGAR.

4. GREEK YOGURT WITH HONEY AND WALNUTS

Ingredients:
- 1/2 cup plain Greek yogurt
- 1 tsp raw honey
- 1 tbsp crushed walnuts

Instructions:
1. Spoon yogurt into a bowl.
2. Drizzle with honey and sprinkle with walnuts.

Nutritional Benefits:
- ⇨ **GREEK YOGURT:** High in PROBIOTICS for GUT HEALTH and PROTEIN for MUSCLE REPAIR.
- ⇨ **HONEY:** Provides NATURAL SWEETNESS and ANTIOXIDANTS.
- ⇨ **WALNUTS:** Rich in OMEGA-3 FATTY ACIDS to reduce INFLAMMATION.

---

5. HARD-BOILED EGGS WITH MUSTARD DIP

Ingredients:
- 2 hard-boiled eggs, peeled
- 1 tsp Dijon mustard
- A pinch of paprika

Instructions:
1. Cut eggs in half and arrange them on a plate.
2. Mix Dijon mustard and paprika in a small bowl for dipping.

Nutritional Benefits:
- ⇨ **EGGS:** Excellent source of PROTEIN and B VITAMINS for ENERGY.
- ⇨ **MUSTARD:** Low in CALORIES and adds FLAVOR without extra FAT.

---

6. APPLE SLICES WITH ALMOND BUTTER

Ingredients:
- 1 medium apple, sliced
- 1 tbsp almond butter

Instructions:
1. Slice the apple and spread almond butter over each slice.

Nutritional Benefits:
- ⇨ **APPLES:** Provide FIBER and NATURAL SUGARS for QUICK ENERGY.
- ⇨ **ALMOND BUTTER:** Adds HEALTHY FATS and PROTEIN to balance BLOOD SUGAR LEVELS.

---

7. EDAMAME WITH SEA SALT

Ingredients:
- 1/2 cup steamed edamame
- A pinch of sea salt

Instructions:
1. Steam edamame until tender, about 5–6 minutes.
2. Sprinkle with sea salt and serve warm or chilled.

Nutritional Benefits:
- ⇨ **EDAMAME:** High in PLANT-BASED PROTEIN and MAGNESIUM for MUSCLE FUNCTION.
- ⇨ **SEA SALT:** Replenishes ELECTROLYTES, helping with HYDRATION.

8. CARROT AND CUCUMBER HUMMUS CUPS

Ingredients:
- 1/2 cup baby carrots
- 1/2 cup cucumber slices
- 2 tbsp hummus

Instructions:
1. Dip carrots and cucumber slices into hummus.

Nutritional Benefits:
- ⇨ **VEGETABLES:** Provide FIBER and ANTIOXIDANTS to reduce INFLAMMATION.
- ⇨ **HUMMUS:** Rich in HEALTHY FATS and PROTEIN for STRESS RELIEF.

---

9. DARK CHOCOLATE ALMOND CLUSTERS

Ingredients (4 clusters):
- 1/4 cup dark chocolate chips
- 1/4 cup almonds
- 1 tbsp unsweetened coconut flakes

Instructions:
1. Melt dark chocolate in the microwave in 30-second intervals, stirring until smooth.
2. Stir in almonds and coconut flakes.
3. Spoon small clusters onto parchment paper and refrigerate for 20 minutes until set.

Nutritional Benefits:
- ⇨ **DARK CHOCOLATE:** Rich in MAGNESIUM and promotes MOOD STABILITY.
- ⇨ **ALMONDS:** Add HEALTHY FATS and PROTEIN for ENERGY.

---

10. CHIA AND COCONUT PUDDING CUPS

Ingredients:
- 3 tbsp chia seeds
- 1/2 cup coconut milk
- 1/2 tsp vanilla extract
- 1 tbsp shredded coconut

Instructions:
1. Mix chia seeds, coconut milk, and vanilla extract in a jar.
2. Stir well to prevent lumps and refrigerate for at least 2 hours (or overnight) until thickened.
3. Top with shredded coconut before serving.

Nutritional Benefits:
- ⇨ **CHIA SEEDS:** Packed with OMEGA-3 FATTY ACIDS, FIBER, and PROTEIN for DIGESTIVE HEALTH and ENERGY STABILITY.
- ⇨ **COCONUT MILK:** Provides HEALTHY FATS for HORMONAL BALANCE and BRAIN FUNCTION.

11. MATCHA ENERGY BITES

Ingredients (3 bites):
- 5 Medjool dates, pitted
- 1 tbsp almond butter
- 1 tsp matcha powder
- 1 tbsp coconut flakes
- 1 tbsp chia seeds

Instructions:
1. Blend dates and almond butter in a food processor until smooth.
2. Add matcha powder, coconut flakes, and chia seeds, then pulse until combined.
3. Roll into 3 small balls and refrigerate for 15–20 minutes before serving.

Nutritional Benefits:
- ⇨ **MATCHA:** Provides ANTIOXIDANTS and boosts ENERGY and FOCUS.
- ⇨ **CHIA SEEDS:** Offer OMEGA-3 FATTY ACIDS and FIBER for DIGESTION.
- ⇨ **COCONUT FLAKES:** Supply HEALTHY FATS for ENERGY and BRAIN HEALTH.

---

12. CUCUMBER AND SMOKED SALMON BITES

Ingredients:
- 6 slices cucumber
- 3 slices smoked salmon
- 2 tbsp cream cheese

Instructions:
1. Spread cream cheese on each cucumber slice.
2. Fold and place smoked salmon on top of half the slices.
3. Cover with the remaining cucumber slices to make mini sandwiches.

Nutritional Benefits:
- ⇨ **SMOKED SALMON**: Rich in OMEGA-3 FATTY ACIDS for INFLAMMATION REDUCTION and BRAIN HEALTH.
- ⇨ **CUCUMBER:** Supports HYDRATION and DETOXIFICATION.
- ⇨ **CREAM CHEESE:** Adds HEALTHY FATS and a CREAMY TEXTURE.

---

13. ROASTED CHICKPEAS WITH SEA SALT AND PAPRIKA

Ingredients:
- 1/2 cup cooked chickpeas (canned, drained, and rinsed)
- 1 tsp olive oil
- 1/2 tsp paprika
- A pinch of sea salt

Instructions:
1. Preheat oven to 400°F (200°C).
2. Toss chickpeas with olive oil, paprika, and sea salt in a bowl.
3. Spread on a baking sheet and roast for 20–25 minutes, shaking halfway through until crispy.

Nutritional Benefits:
- ⇨ **CHICKPEAS:** Provide FIBER and PROTEIN to CURB CRAVINGS and MAINTAIN ENERGY BALANCE.
- ⇨ **PAPRIKA:** Adds ANTIOXIDANTS and may BOOST METABOLISM.
- ⇨ **OLIVE OIL:** Offers HEALTHY MONOUNSATURATED FATS.

14. TURMERIC ROASTED CASHEWS

Ingredients:
- 1/2 cup raw cashews
- 1/2 tsp turmeric powder
- 1 tsp coconut oil, melted
- A pinch of black pepper

Instructions:
1. Preheat oven to 350°F (175°C).
2. Toss cashews with turmeric, coconut oil, and black pepper in a bowl.
3. Spread cashews on a baking sheet and roast for 8–10 minutes, stirring occasionally.

Nutritional Benefits:
- ⇨ **CASHEWS:** High in MAGNESIUM and HEALTHY FATS to support MUSCLE FUNCTION and ENERGY.
- ⇨ **TURMERIC:** Contains ANTI-INFLAMMATORY PROPERTIES enhanced by BLACK PEPPER for better absorption of CURCUMIN.
- ⇨ **COCONUT OIL:** Provides MCTs (MEDIUM-CHAIN TRIGLYCERIDES) for QUICK ENERGY.

SMOOTHIES FOR STRESS RELIEF AND HORMONAL BALANCE

1. GREEN DETOX SMOOTHIE

Ingredients:
- 1 cup spinach
- 1/2 cucumber, peeled and chopped
- 1/2 green apple, chopped
- 1/2 avocado
- 1 tbsp chia seeds
- 1 cup coconut water
- Juice of 1/2 lemon

Instructions:
1. Blend all ingredients until smooth.
2. Serve immediately.

Nutritional Benefits:
- ⇨ **SPINACH:** Rich in MAGNESIUM, reduces MUSCLE TENSION and promotes RELAXATION.
- ⇨ **CHIA SEEDS:** High in OMEGA-3s and FIBER to stabilize BLOOD SUGAR.
- ⇨ **AVOCADO:** Packed with HEALTHY FATS to support HORMONE PRODUCTION.

2. GOLDEN TURMERIC SMOOTHIE

Ingredients:
- 1 cup almond milk (unsweetened)
- 1/2 banana
- 1 tsp turmeric powder
- 1/2 tsp cinnamon
- 1/2 tsp ginger powder
- 1 tsp honey
- 1 tbsp almond butter

Instructions:
1. Blend all ingredients until creamy.
2. Serve chilled or warm for a comforting drink.

Nutritional Benefits:
- ⇨ **TURMERIC:** Powerful ANTI-INFLAMMATORY and supports ADRENAL HEALTH.
- ⇨ **GINGER:** Improves DIGESTION and reduces NAUSEA.
- ⇨ **ALMOND BUTTER:** Provides PROTEIN and HEALTHY FATS for sustained ENERGY.

3. BERRY ANTIOXIDANT BLAST

Ingredients:
- 1/2 cup blueberries
- 1/2 cup strawberries
- 1/2 cup Greek yogurt
- 1 tbsp flaxseeds
- 1 cup almond milk

Instructions:
1. Blend all ingredients until smooth.
2. Add ice cubes if desired and blend again.

Nutritional Benefits:
- ⇨ **BERRIES:** High in ANTIOXIDANTS to combat OXIDATIVE STRESS.
- ⇨ **FLAXSEEDS:** Provide LIGNANS and OMEGA-3s for HORMONE BALANCE.
- ⇨ **GREEK YOGURT:** Supports GUT HEALTH with PROBIOTICS.

---

4. COCONUT MATCHA ENERGY SMOOTHIE

Ingredients:
- 1 cup coconut milk
- 1/2 frozen banana
- 1 tsp matcha powder
- 1 tbsp chia seeds
- 1 tsp honey

Instructions:
1. Blend all ingredients until creamy.
2. Serve cold.

Nutritional Benefits:
- ⇨ **MATCHA:** Provides GENTLE CAFFEINE for FOCUS without JITTERS.
- ⇨ **CHIA SEEDS:** Fiber-rich for BLOOD SUGAR CONTROL.
- ⇨ **COCONUT MILK:** Source of HEALTHY FATS for ENERGY and SATIETY.

---

5. TROPICAL STRESS-RELIEF SMOOTHIE

Ingredients:
- 1/2 cup mango
- 1/2 cup pineapple
- 1/2 banana
- 1 cup coconut water
- 1 tbsp hemp seeds

Instructions:
- Blend all ingredients until smooth.
- Serve chilled.

Nutritional Benefits:
- ⇨ **MANGO & PINEAPPLE:** High in VITAMIN C to lower CORTISOL.
- ⇨ **HEMP SEEDS:** Contain OMEGA-3s and MAGNESIUM to CALM the nervous system.
- ⇨ **COCONUT WATER:** Provides ELECTROLYTES for HYDRATION.

6. PROTEIN POWER CACAO SMOOTHIE

Ingredients:
- 1 cup almond milk
- 1 scoop chocolate protein powder
- 1 tbsp cacao powder
- 1/2 banana
- 1 tbsp peanut butter

Instructions:
1. Blend all ingredients until creamy.
2. Serve with ice cubes for a refreshing drink.

Nutritional Benefits:
- ⇨ **CACAO POWDER:** Rich in MAGNESIUM and MOOD-BOOSTING COMPOUNDS.
- ⇨ **PROTEIN POWDER:** Supports MUSCLE REPAIR and BLOOD SUGAR STABILITY.
- ⇨ **PEANUT BUTTER:** Healthy fats for ENERGY and SATIETY.

7. SAVORY AVOCADO & SPINACH SMOOTHIE

Ingredients:
- 1 cup spinach
- 1/2 avocado
- 1/4 cup cucumber
- 1 tbsp lemon juice
- 1/2 tsp sea salt
- 1 cup water

Instructions:
1. Blend all ingredients until smooth.
2. Serve chilled.

Nutritional Benefits:
- ⇨ **AVOCADO:** Healthy fats for HORMONE SUPPORT.
- ⇨ **CUCUMBER:** Hydrating and rich in ANTIOXIDANTS.
- ⇨ **LEMON JUICE:** Supports DETOXIFICATION and VITAMIN C levels.

8. SPICY TOMATO DETOX SMOOTHIE

Ingredients:
- 1 cup tomato juice
- 1/4 cucumber
- 1/4 red bell pepper
- 1 tbsp lemon juice
- A pinch of cayenne pepper

Instructions:
1. Blend all ingredients until smooth.
2. Serve immediately.

Nutritional Benefits:
- ⇨ **TOMATOES:** Rich in LYCOPENE, which fights INFLAMMATION.
- ⇨ **CAYENNE PEPPER:** Stimulates CIRCULATION and boosts METABOLISM.
- ⇨ **BELL PEPPER:** High in VITAMIN C for IMMUNITY SUPPORT.

9. CREAMY AVOCADO & CILANTRO SMOOTHIE

Ingredients:
- 1/2 avocado
- 1/2 cup cilantro
- 1/2 cucumber
- 1/2 cup Greek yogurt
- Juice of 1 lime

Instructions:
1. Blend until smooth and creamy.
2. Serve chilled.

Nutritional Benefits:
- ⇨ **CILANTRO:** Natural DETOXIFIER that helps ELIMINATE TOXINS.
- ⇨ **AVOCADO:** Healthy fats to STABILIZE MOOD and ENERGY.
- ⇨ **GREEK YOGURT:** PROBIOTICS for DIGESTION and IMMUNITY.

---

10. CARROT-GINGER IMMUNITY BOOSTER

Ingredients:
- 1 cup carrot juice
- 1/2 orange
- 1/2 tsp ginger
- 1/2 tsp turmeric
- 1 tsp honey

Instructions:
1. Blend all ingredients until smooth.
2. Serve cold.

Nutritional Benefits:
- ⇨ **CARROTS:** Rich in BETA-CAROTENE to support IMMUNE FUNCTION.
- ⇨ **GINGER & TURMERIC:** Reduce INFLAMMATION and aid DIGESTION.
- ⇨ **HONEY:** Provides NATURAL SWEETNESS and ANTIBACTERIAL properties.

---

11. MINTY CUCUMBER REFRESHER

Ingredients:
- 1 cup cucumber, peeled and chopped
- 1/2 cup fresh mint leaves
- 1/2 lime, juiced
- 1 cup coconut water
- 1 tsp honey (optional)

Instructions:
1. Blend all ingredients until smooth.
2. Serve chilled with ice.

Nutritional Benefits:
- ⇨ **CUCUMBER:** Hydrating and RICH IN ANTIOXIDANTS.
- ⇨ **MINT:** Supports DIGESTION and reduces BLOATING.
- ⇨ **COCONUT WATER:** Restores ELECTROLYTES and HYDRATES.

12. CHERRY VANILLA DREAM

Ingredients:
- 1 cup frozen cherries
- 1/2 frozen banana
- 1 cup almond milk
- 1/2 tsp vanilla extract
- 1 tbsp chia seeds

Instructions:
1. Blend all ingredients until creamy.
2. Serve immediately.

Nutritional Benefits:
- ⇨ **CHERRIES:** Rich in MELATONIN for BETTER SLEEP.
- ⇨ **CHIA SEEDS:** High in FIBER and OMEGA-3s for HORMONE BALANCE.
- ⇨ **VANILLA:** Adds NATURAL SWEETNESS and CALMING AROMA.

13. CHOCOLATE AVOCADO MOUSSE SMOOTHIE

Ingredients:
- 1/2 avocado
- 1 tbsp cacao powder
- 1 cup almond milk
- 1 tbsp maple syrup
- 1/2 tsp cinnamon

Instructions:
1. Blend until smooth and creamy.
2. Serve as a smoothie or dessert.

Nutritional Benefits:
- ⇨ **CACAO:** Boosts MOOD and ENERGY with MAGNESIUM.
- ⇨ **AVOCADO:** Healthy FATS for HORMONAL HEALTH.
- ⇨ **CINNAMON:** Stabilizes BLOOD SUGAR.

14. SPICY MANGO CHILI SMOOTHIE

Ingredients:
- 1 cup mango
- 1/2 cup coconut milk
- 1/4 tsp chili powder
- 1/2 lime, juiced
- 1 tsp honey

Instructions:
1. Blend all ingredients until smooth.
2. Serve immediately.

Nutritional Benefits:
- ⇨ **MANGO:** Rich in VITAMIN C to lower CORTISOL.
- ⇨ **CHILI POWDER:** Boosts METABOLISM and reduces INFLAMMATION.
- ⇨ **COCONUT MILK:** Healthy FATS for ENERGY.

15. PEACH GINGER IMMUNE BOOSTER

Ingredients:
1 cup frozen peaches
1/2 tsp grated ginger
1 cup coconut water
1 tbsp flaxseeds
1 tsp honey

Instructions:
Blend until smooth and serve cold.

Nutritional Benefits:
- ⇨ **PEACHES:** Rich in ANTIOXIDANTS and VITAMIN C.
- ⇨ **GINGER:** Anti-inflammatory and supports DIGESTION.
- ⇨ **FLAXSEEDS:** Hormone-regulating OMEGA-3s.

16. APPLE PIE SMOOTHIE

Ingredients:
- 1 cup apple, chopped
- 1/2 frozen banana
- 1/2 tsp cinnamon
- 1/2 cup oat milk
- 1 tbsp almond butter

Instructions:
1. Blend until creamy and enjoy chilled.

Nutritional Benefits:
- ⇨ **APPLE:** Rich in FIBER to support DIGESTION.
- ⇨ **CINNAMON:** Balances BLOOD SUGAR and fights INFLAMMATION.
- ⇨ **ALMOND BUTTER:** Provides PROTEIN and HEALTHY FATS.

17. BLUEBERRY LAVENDER CALMING SMOOTHIE

Ingredients:
- 1/2 cup blueberries
- 1 cup almond milk
- 1 tsp dried lavender flowers
- 1 tbsp honey
- 1/2 tsp vanilla extract

Instructions:
1. Blend until smooth and strain if desired.

Nutritional Benefits:
- ⇨ **BLUEBERRIES:** Packed with ANTIOXIDANTS to reduce OXIDATIVE STRESS.
- ⇨ **LAVENDER:** Calming effect on the NERVOUS SYSTEM.
- ⇨ **HONEY:** Natural SWEETENER with ANTI-INFLAMMATORY properties.

18. PINEAPPLE CUCUMBER GREEN SMOOTHIE

Ingredients:
- 1/2 cup pineapple
- 1/2 cucumber
- 1/2 cup kale or spinach
- 1 cup coconut water
- 1 tbsp chia seeds

Instructions:
1. Blend until smooth and serve immediately.

Nutritional Benefits:
- ⇨ **PINEAPPLE:** Rich in BROMELAIN for DIGESTION and ANTI-INFLAMMATORY support.
- ⇨ **KALE:** High in VITAMIN C and MAGNESIUM for STRESS RELIEF.
- ⇨ **COCONUT WATER:** HYDRATES and replenishes ELECTROLYTES.

---

19. STRAWBERRY CREAM SMOOTHIE

Ingredients:
- 1 cup strawberries
- 1/2 frozen banana
- 1 cup oat milk
- 1 tbsp cashew butter

Instructions:
1. Blend all ingredients until creamy and smooth.

Nutritional Benefits:
- ⇨ **STRAWBERRIES:** High in VITAMIN C for IMMUNITY and COLLAGEN PRODUCTION.
- ⇨ **CASHEW BUTTER:** Provides PROTEIN and HEALTHY FATS.
- ⇨ **OAT MILK:** Naturally CALMING and rich in FIBER.

---

20. AVOCADO-CACAO ENERGY SHAKE

Ingredients:
- 1/2 avocado
- 1 cup almond milk
- 1 tbsp cacao powder
- 1 tbsp honey
- 1/2 tsp maca powder

Instructions:
1. Blend until smooth and creamy.
2. Serve chilled.

Nutritional Benefits:
- ⇨ **CACAO:** Supports MOOD and ENERGY with MAGNESIUM.
- ⇨ **MACA POWDER:** Hormone BALANCER and ENERGY BOOSTER.
- ⇨ **AVOCADO:** Healthy FATS for SUSTAINED ENERGY.

QUICK AND EASY MEAL PREP TIPS

Batch Cooking for Stress-Free Meals

Prepare large portions of QUINOA, BROWN RICE, or ROASTED VEGETABLES at the start of the week. Store them in GLASS CONTAINERS to keep them fresh and ready for use.

Freezer-Friendly Options

Freeze individual servings of SOUPS, CURRIES, and SMOOTHIE PACKS for quick grab-and-go meals during busy days.

Overnight Prep for Breakfasts

Assemble OVERNIGHT OATS, CHIA PUDDINGS, and SMOOTHIE JARS the night before to save time in the morning.

Portioning Snacks in Advance

Pre-pack NUTS, SEEDS, and ENERGY BALLS in reusable bags or jars to have healthy snacks within reach at all times.

Building Balanced Plates

When assembling meals, focus on combining a LEAN PROTEIN, a HEALTHY FAT, and a COMPLEX CARBOHYDRATE. This trio helps to SUSTAIN ENERGY and REDUCE CRAVINGS.

Keep a Weekly Plan

Create a WEEKLY MEAL SCHEDULE to stay organized and avoid reaching for PROCESSED FOODS in moments of stress.

These recipes and strategies provide a STRUCTURED YET FLEXIBLE framework for balancing cortisol levels through nutrition. By integrating these nutrient-dense meals and snacks into daily routines, it becomes easier to FUEL THE BODY, REDUCE INFLAMMATION, and RESTORE HORMONAL BALANCE.

CHAPTER 4: THE 7-DAY RESET PLAN

Your body is constantly working to maintain balance, but the demands of modern life—stress, poor eating habits, and environmental toxins—can throw that balance off course. *The 7-Day Reset Plan* is a structured yet flexible roadmap designed to help you *recharge, rejuvenate*, and *reconnect* with your body's natural rhythms.

This plan isn't about deprivation or extreme dieting; instead, it focuses on *nourishing foods, gentle movement*, and *mindfulness practices* to support your body's natural ability to *heal and thrive*. Each day introduces *simple, purposeful actions* that build sustainable habits, allowing you to experience both *physical vitality* and *emotional clarity*.

Over the course of seven days, you'll explore *balanced meal plans, stress-relief techniques*, and *movement practices* designed to energize your mornings, *sustain focus* throughout the day, and *promote deep relaxation* in the evening. Paired with *journaling prompts* to deepen self-awareness, this program is more than just a diet—it's an *invitation to reset your habits, revitalize your energy*, and *rediscover balance*.

By the end of this week, you'll not only feel physically lighter but also mentally clearer, ready to move forward with *confidence* and *purpose*.

4.1 HOW TO START YOUR DETOX JOURNEY

Embarking on a DETOX JOURNEY can feel both exhilarating and overwhelming. It's not just about eliminating certain foods or adopting new habits—it's about reshaping your mindset, honoring your body, and embracing a process of renewal. The first week is often the most pivotal, as it sets the tone for how well your body adapts to the shift. This section provides a clear blueprint for SETTING UP YOUR DAILY ROUTINE and OVERCOMING CHALLENGES so that your detox journey begins with confidence and clarity.

SETTING UP YOUR DAILY ROUTINE: MORNING, AFTERNOON, AND EVENING PRACTICES

Your daily routine is the foundation of a successful detox. By aligning your habits with your goals, you create structure and consistency that reinforces your commitment. Think of your routine as a RHYTHMIC FLOW, not a rigid schedule, allowing space for flexibility and self-compassion.

MORNING PRACTICES: AWAKEN AND ALIGN

Mornings are a POWERFUL RESET POINT. They set the emotional and physical tone for the rest of the day.

1. **Hydrate Immediately** – Start your day with a GLASS OF WARM LEMON WATER. This simple ritual stimulates digestion, FLUSHES TOXINS, and rehydrates your cells after hours of fasting during sleep. Add a pinch of HIMALAYAN SALT for trace minerals or a slice of GINGER for an anti-inflammatory boost.

2. **Gentle Movement** – Engage in STRETCHING, YOGA FLOWS, or a brief MORNING WALK. Movement activates circulation, AWAKENS YOUR LYMPHATIC SYSTEM, and primes your metabolism. Even five minutes of intentional breathing can REDUCE CORTISOL LEVELS and promote clarity.

3. **Mindful Reflection** – Journaling or MEDITATION helps center your thoughts. Take a moment to write down a DAILY AFFIRMATION or a goal for your detox journey. Focus on phrases like: "I HONOR MY BODY'S ABILITY TO HEAL."

4. **Nourishing Breakfast** – Choose a meal rich in FIBER, HEALTHY FATS, and PROTEIN to stabilize blood sugar and sustain energy. Options might include a CHIA SEED PUDDING, a GREEN SMOOTHIE, or AVOCADO TOAST with a sprinkle of HEMP SEEDS.

AFTERNOON PRACTICES: FUEL AND REBALANCE
The afternoon often brings the HIGHEST ENERGY DEMANDS and, for many, the most cravings. Structuring this part of the day ensures you stay grounded and focused.

1. **Midday Check-In** – Pause for a DEEP-BREATHING EXERCISE to break mental patterns of stress or fatigue. Try the 4-7-8 TECHNIQUE: inhale for 4 seconds, hold for 7, exhale for 8. This process can CALM THE NERVOUS SYSTEM and prevent stress eating.
2. **Smart Snacking** – Keep a selection of NUTRIENT-DENSE SNACKS within reach. Opt for ALMOND BUTTER WITH APPLE SLICES, EDAMAME WITH SEA SALT, or CHIA PUDDING. These snacks prevent energy crashes while maintaining BLOOD SUGAR STABILITY.
3. **Movement Break** – Incorporate LIGHT ACTIVITY, whether it's a brisk walk, DESK STRETCHES, or YOGA POSES. This not only STIMULATES DIGESTION but also helps to release ENDORPHINS, lifting your mood.
4. **Herbal Support** – Sip on HERBAL TEAS that support detoxification, such as DANDELION ROOT, PEPPERMINT, or GINGER TURMERIC BLENDS. These teas promote LIVER FUNCTION, soothe digestion, and provide ANTI-INFLAMMATORY BENEFITS.

EVENING PRACTICES: UNWIND AND RESTORE
Evenings are about RESTORATION. It's the time to RELEASE STRESS, REJUVENATE YOUR SYSTEM, and PREPARE FOR DEEP SLEEP.

1. **Light Dinner** – Focus on EASILY DIGESTIBLE MEALS such as soups, stews, or VEGETABLE STIR-FRIES. Avoid heavy or processed foods, which can interfere with detoxification overnight.
2. **Detox Baths** – Take a warm bath with EPSOM SALTS and LAVENDER ESSENTIAL OIL. The magnesium in Epsom salts aids in MUSCLE RELAXATION and supports detox pathways, while lavender calms the mind.
3. **Screen-Free Hour** – Limit exposure to blue light from devices, as it can disrupt MELATONIN PRODUCTION. Instead, read, meditate, or listen to calming music.
4. **Gratitude Journaling** – Reflect on POSITIVE MOMENTS from the day. Write about any changes you've noticed—improved digestion, clearer skin, or a lighter mood. Gratitude can reinforce EMOTIONAL RESILIENCE throughout your detox.

OVERCOMING COMMON CHALLENGES IN THE FIRST WEEK
The first week of detoxing isn't always smooth. Your body may respond with DETOX SYMPTOMS such as fatigue, headaches, or irritability as it eliminates built-up toxins. These experiences are TEMPORARY and can be managed with preparation and mindfulness.

CRAVINGS AND HUNGER
Cravings often arise when your body is adjusting to a lower intake of SUGAR or PROCESSED FOODS. Combat this by:

- Drinking water infused with LEMON or MINT to curb cravings.
- Opting for snacks high in FIBER and PROTEIN, such as ROASTED CHICKPEAS or GREEK YOGURT.
- Distracting yourself with ACTIVITY, whether it's walking, journaling, or STRETCHING.

ENERGY DIPS AND FATIGUE
Low energy is common as your body shifts from burning CARBOHYDRATES to using FATS for fuel. Restore balance by:

- Eating SMALL, FREQUENT MEALS rich in HEALTHY FATS and COMPLEX CARBS.
- Prioritizing SLEEP HYGIENE—set a consistent bedtime and avoid caffeine after 2 p.m.
- Incorporating ADAPTOGENIC HERBS like ASHWAGANDHA or HOLY BASIL to support your adrenal system.

DIGESTIVE UPSET
Bloating or irregularity can occur when your body adjusts to HIGHER FIBER INTAKE. Ease this with:
- Drinking WARM HERBAL TEAS like PEPPERMINT or FENNEL.
- Consuming PROBIOTIC-RICH FOODS such as KIMCHI, YOGURT, or SAUERKRAUT.
- Moving gently—try TWISTING YOGA POSES to stimulate digestion.

MOOD SWINGS AND IRRITABILITY
Shifting your diet affects HORMONES and NEUROTRANSMITTERS, sometimes leading to EMOTIONAL UPS AND DOWNS. Stabilize your mood by:
- Journaling daily reflections and tracking emotional patterns.
- Practicing MEDITATION or DEEP BREATHING exercises to regain focus.
- Eating foods rich in MAGNESIUM and B VITAMINS like LEAFY GREENS, NUTS, and SEEDS.

SLEEP DISTURBANCES
Detoxing can temporarily disrupt SLEEP CYCLES. Enhance restfulness by:
- Drinking CHAMOMILE TEA before bed to calm the nervous system.
- Diffusing LAVENDER ESSENTIAL OIL in your bedroom for AROMATHERAPY.
- Listening to WHITE NOISE or NATURE SOUNDS to ease into sleep.

Your detox journey begins with intention and routine. By honoring your MORNING RITUALS, AFTERNOON RESETS, and EVENING WIND-DOWNS, you create a sustainable rhythm that supports both PHYSICAL HEALING and EMOTIONAL BALANCE. This foundation ensures that the first week is not just about ENDURANCE but about TRANSFORMATION.

4.2 THE 7-DAY PLAN

The 7-DAY RESET PLAN is designed to guide you through a structured yet flexible framework to help your body and mind rebalance, recharge, and realign. This plan blends NOURISHING MEALS, GENTLE MOVEMENT, and MINDFULNESS PRACTICES to create a foundation for sustainable wellness. Each day introduces small, intentional changes that build momentum and reinforce HEALTHY HABITS.

By the end of this week, you may notice increased energy, mental clarity, and a greater sense of CALM. The focus is on progress, not perfection—allow yourself grace as you navigate the shifts and discoveries that emerge along the way.

DAY 1: AWAKENING AWARENESS
Focus: LAYING THE FOUNDATION

Meals and Snacks
- **Breakfast:** AVOCADO TOAST WITH HEMP SEEDS – A slice of sprouted-grain toast topped with mashed avocado, a sprinkle of HEMP SEEDS, and a dash of LEMON JUICE.
- **Mid-Morning Snack:** CHIA PUDDING WITH ALMOND BUTTER – Prepared with COCONUT MILK, CHIA SEEDS, and a drizzle of ALMOND BUTTER.
- **Lunch:** DETOX KALE SALAD WITH LEMON-TAHINI DRESSING – Fresh kale, CUCUMBER, BEETS, and QUINOA, tossed with a CREAMY TAHINI-LEMON DRESSING.
- **Afternoon Snack:** CARROT STICKS AND HUMMUS – Provides FIBER and HEALTHY FATS to curb cravings.
- **Dinner:** TURMERIC LENTIL SOUP – Made with CARROTS, ONIONS, COCONUT MILK, and TURMERIC for an ANTI-INFLAMMATORY BOOST.

Movement and Relaxation
- **Morning Yoga Flow:** A gentle 10-MINUTE SEQUENCE to STIMULATE CIRCULATION.
- **Evening Stretch Routine:** Focus on HIP-OPENERS and SPINAL TWISTS to release tension.

Journaling Prompt: WHAT INSPIRED YOU TO START THIS DETOX? Reflect on your intentions and emotional readiness.

DAY 2: DETOX AND RELEASE
Focus: SUPPORTING DIGESTION AND CIRCULATION

Meals and Snacks
- **Breakfast:** GREEN SMOOTHIE WITH SPINACH, BANANA, AND SPIRULINA – Boosts DETOXIFICATION ENZYMES.
- **Mid-Morning Snack:** HARD-BOILED EGGS WITH PAPRIKA – Offers PROTEIN to sustain energy.
- **Lunch:** STUFFED BELL PEPPERS WITH QUINOA AND BLACK BEANS – Rich in FIBER and ANTIOXIDANTS.
- **Afternoon Snack:** EDAMAME WITH SEA SALT – A source of PLANT-BASED PROTEIN.
- **Dinner:** BAKED SALMON WITH STEAMED ASPARAGUS AND LEMON BUTTER SAUCE – Packed with OMEGA-3 FATTY ACIDS.

Movement and Relaxation
- **Midday Walk:** Spend 20 minutes outside to BOOST VITAMIN D and REDUCE STRESS.
- **Evening Guided Meditation:** Focus on DEEP BREATHING and GRATITUDE PRACTICES.

Journaling Prompt: WHAT EMOTIONS SURFACED TODAY? Write down any patterns or shifts you noticed.

DAY 3: GROUNDING AND STABILITY
Focus: BALANCING ENERGY AND MOOD

Meals and Snacks
- **Breakfast:** OVERNIGHT OATS WITH CHIA SEEDS AND ALMOND MILK – Prepares the body for SUSTAINED ENERGY.
- **Mid-Morning Snack:** CUCUMBER SLICES WITH GUACAMOLE – Refreshing and HYDRATING.
- **Lunch:** ZUCCHINI NOODLES WITH AVOCADO PESTO – Provides HEALTHY FATS and FIBER.
- **Afternoon Snack:** ROASTED CHICKPEAS WITH PAPRIKA – Crunchy and SATISFYING.
- **Dinner:** CAULIFLOWER STIR-FRY WITH TOFU AND GINGER – Rich in PROTEIN and ANTI-INFLAMMATORY PROPERTIES.

Movement and Relaxation
- **Morning Walk or Jog:** Spend 15–20 minutes in NATURE.
- **Evening Foam Rolling Session:** Release MUSCLE TENSION and IMPROVE FLEXIBILITY.

Journaling Prompt: WHAT ARE YOU MOST GRATEFUL FOR TODAY? Reflect on small victories.

DAY 4: REJUVENATION AND RENEWAL
Focus: DEEPENING DETOX PATHWAYS

Meals and Snacks
- **Breakfast:** SMOOTHIE BOWL WITH MIXED BERRIES AND COCONUT FLAKES.
- **Mid-Morning Snack:** GREEK YOGURT WITH WALNUTS AND HONEY.
- **Lunch:** RAINBOW BUDDHA BOWL WITH TAHINI DRESSING.
- **Afternoon Snack:** APPLE SLICES WITH ALMOND BUTTER.
- **Dinner:** STUFFED SWEET POTATO WITH BLACK BEANS AND AVOCADO.

Movement and Relaxation
- **Morning Pilates Session:** Focus on CORE STRENGTH.
- **Evening Epsom Salt Bath:** Add LAVENDER ESSENTIAL OIL for deeper relaxation.

Journaling Prompt: WHAT HAS BEEN THE MOST CHALLENGING PART OF THIS DETOX SO FAR? Explore ways to overcome those hurdles.

DAY 5: STRENGTH AND ENERGY

Focus: REVITALIZING THE BODY AND SUSTAINING ENERGY

Meals and Snacks
- **Breakfast:** PROTEIN SMOOTHIE WITH BANANA AND PEANUT BUTTER.
- **Mid-Morning Snack:** DARK CHOCOLATE ALMOND CLUSTERS.
- **Lunch:** QUINOA AND CHICKPEA SALAD WITH LEMON VINAIGRETTE.
- **Afternoon Snack:** SEAWEED SNACKS AND CASHEWS.
- **Dinner:** GRILLED CHICKEN WITH ROASTED BRUSSELS SPROUTS.

Movement and Relaxation
- **Morning Cardio Session:** Boosts METABOLISM.
- **Evening Gentle Stretching Routine:** Focus on HIPS and HAMSTRINGS.

Journaling Prompt: WHAT DOES FEELING STRONG MEAN TO YOU?

DAY 6: CLARITY AND FOCUS

Focus: ENHANCING MENTAL SHARPNESS

Meals and Snacks
- **Breakfast:** MATCHA ENERGY BITES WITH COCONUT FLAKES.
- **Mid-Morning Snack:** TURMERIC ROASTED CASHEWS.
- **Lunch:** SPINACH AND MUSHROOM OMELET.
- **Afternoon Snack:** GREEN JUICE WITH CELERY AND GINGER.
- **Dinner:** VEGETABLE CURRY WITH BROWN RICE.

Movement and Relaxation
- **Morning Yoga Session:** Promotes MENTAL CLARITY.
- **Evening Breathing Practice:** Focus on STRESS RELEASE.

Journaling Prompt: WHAT ARE YOU LEARNING ABOUT YOUR BODY THIS WEEK?

DAY 7: REFLECTION AND RENEWAL

Focus: CELEBRATING PROGRESS AND SETTING INTENTIONS

Meals and Snacks
- **Breakfast:** CHIA AND COCONUT PUDDING.
- **Mid-Morning Snack:** MIXED NUTS AND BERRIES.
- **Lunch:** AVOCADO AND SEA SALT RICE CAKES.
- **Afternoon Snack:** CUCUMBER AND SMOKED SALMON BITES.
- **Dinner:** LENTIL STEW WITH KALE AND CARROTS.

Movement and Relaxation
- **Morning Meditation:** Focus on SELF-AWARENESS.
- **Evening Gratitude Walk:** Reflect on achievements.

Journaling Prompt: WHAT HABITS DO YOU WANT TO CONTINUE?

Conclusion to Chapter 4: The 7-Day Reset Plan

Completing the 7-DAY RESET PLAN is more than a personal accomplishment—it's a FOUNDATION FOR LASTING TRANSFORMATION. This week has equipped you with tools to NOURISH YOUR BODY, CALM YOUR MIND, and BOOST YOUR ENERGY naturally. You've learned to listen to your body's signals, PRIORITIZE SELF-CARE, and create routines that support WELLNESS.

As you move forward, carry the lessons and practices you've gained into your daily life. Keep experimenting with RECIPES, MOVEMENT STYLES, and MINDFULNESS TECHNIQUES that resonate with you. Small, consistent steps lead to BIG, SUSTAINABLE CHANGES.

Remember that SELF-CARE ISN'T A LUXURY—IT'S A NECESSITY. Use this reset as a LAUNCHPAD to continue building a lifestyle rooted in BALANCE, VITALITY, and CLARITY. Your journey doesn't end here; it's just the beginning of FEELING YOUR BEST SELF.

CHAPTER 5: THE 14-DAY TRANSFORMATION PLAN

Transformation isn't about quick fixes—it's about *lasting change*. The *14-Day Transformation Plan* is designed to guide you through a *deeper reset*, moving beyond surface-level habits to create a *lifestyle shift* rooted in *balance* and *sustainability*. Over the next two weeks, you'll build upon the foundation set in earlier stages and explore strategies that nurture *physical health*, *emotional well-being*, and *mental resilience*.

The first week focuses on *stability*, helping you establish routines that support *nutrition*, *movement*, and *sleep*. It's about *structure*—building habits that feel *sustainable*, not overwhelming. Then, as you move into Week Two, the focus expands to *advanced strategies*. You'll learn how to *reduce mental stress*, *strengthen relationships*, and *embrace creativity* as tools for *growth*.

This chapter doesn't just prescribe routines—it *empowers you* to *adapt the plan* to fit your *unique goals*. Whether you're looking to *refocus priorities*, *boost energy*, or *cultivate joy*, this plan meets you where you are and helps you *elevate* your journey. Think of these 14 days as a *springboard* for long-term transformation—one that leaves you feeling *clearer*, *stronger*, and more *connected* to yourself.

5.1 WEEK ONE: BUILDING THE FOUNDATION

LAYING THE GROUNDWORK FOR LASTING CHANGE

The first week of the 14-DAY TRANSFORMATION PLAN sets the tone for meaningful and sustainable change. It's not about perfection—it's about MOMENTUM. The goal is to BUILD HABITS that promote NUTRITION, MOVEMENT, and RESTORATIVE SLEEP while cultivating EMOTIONAL RESILIENCE.

This initial phase isn't just about following steps; it's about creating a STRUCTURE that supports your well-being. Think of this week as the FOUNDATION—the stronger it is, the easier it will be to EXPAND AND ADAPT in the days ahead.

By the end of Week One, you'll feel more IN TUNE WITH YOUR BODY, more ENERGIZED, and more CAPABLE of handling stress. You'll not only notice physical changes but also a MENTAL SHIFT that helps you stay focused on your goals without feeling RESTRICTED or OVERWHELMED.

SOLIDIFYING NEW HABITS FOR NUTRITION

Food is FUEL, but it's also INFORMATION. Every bite you take SIGNALS something to your body—whether it's energy, nourishment, or inflammation. The first step in building a NUTRITIONAL FOUNDATION is learning how to LISTEN TO YOUR BODY'S CUES and RESPOND WITH INTENTION.

Key Strategies for Nutritional Success:

- **Simplify Your Plate:** Focus on WHOLE FOODS—lean proteins, colorful vegetables, and HEALTHY FATS. Avoid over-complicating meals; SIMPLICITY reduces DECISION FATIGUE.
- **Front-Load Nutrition:** Begin your day with a HIGH-PROTEIN BREAKFAST to STABILIZE BLOOD SUGAR and reduce CRAVINGS later. For example, scrambled eggs with spinach and avocado or a protein smoothie with almond butter and berries.
- **Hydration Habits:** Drink 16 OUNCES OF WATER as soon as you wake up. This KICKSTARTS DIGESTION and REPLENISHES CELLS. Add a SPLASH OF LEMON for extra ALKALINITY.
- **Balanced Snacks:** Keep ENERGY LEVELS STEADY by pairing PROTEIN with FIBER-RICH CARBOHYDRATES. Examples include APPLE SLICES WITH ALMOND BUTTER or GREEK YOGURT WITH WALNUTS AND HONEY.
- **Meal Planning Basics:** Dedicate 10 MINUTES EACH NIGHT to reviewing the next day's meals. Prep vegetables, soak grains, or portion out snacks. PREPARATION ELIMINATES EXCUSES.

Why It Works:

This approach doesn't just IMPROVE METABOLISM—it reduces INFLAMMATION, enhances DIGESTION, and supports HORMONAL BALANCE. By prioritizing CONSISTENCY over PERFECTION, you'll avoid burnout and create SUSTAINABLE PATTERNS.

MOVEMENT: BUILDING STRENGTH AND FLEXIBILITY

Movement isn't just about BURNING CALORIES. It's about BUILDING ENERGY and RESILIENCE. In Week One, the focus is on CONSISTENT ACTIVITY rather than intensity. The goal is to make movement a NON-NEGOTIABLE PART OF YOUR ROUTINE.

Daily Movement Practices:

- **Morning Activation (10 Minutes):** Start each day with DYNAMIC STRETCHES like CAT-COW STRETCHES, HIP OPENERS, and ARM CIRCLES. This WAKES UP THE BODY and BOOSTS CIRCULATION.
- **Midday Energy Boost (15 Minutes):** Incorporate BODYWEIGHT EXERCISES—squats, lunges, and planks—during a lunch break. These movements RELEASE ENDORPHINS and REDUCE AFTERNOON FATIGUE.
- **Evening Relaxation (10 Minutes):** End the day with GENTLE YOGA or FOAM ROLLING to UNWIND MUSCLES and PREPARE THE BODY FOR REST. Focus on DEEP BREATHING to LOWER CORTISOL LEVELS.

Why It Works:

Consistent, LOW-IMPACT MOVEMENT reduces MUSCLE TENSION, improves POSTURE, and supports EMOTIONAL REGULATION. Pairing activity with BREATHWORK amplifies these effects, helping the body RELEASE STRESS and RESTORE BALANCE.

PRIORITIZING RESTORATIVE SLEEP

Sleep is often overlooked, but it's the CORNERSTONE of any transformation. Poor sleep disrupts HORMONES, slows METABOLISM, and triggers CRAVINGS. Week One focuses on creating a SLEEP-FRIENDLY ENVIRONMENT and establishing BEDTIME RITUALS that signal the body to UNWIND.

Key Sleep Strategies:

- **Set a Schedule:** Go to bed and wake up at the SAME TIME EACH DAY to REGULATE CIRCADIAN RHYTHMS. Consistency strengthens the SLEEP-WAKE CYCLE.
- **Dim the Lights:** Reduce BLUE LIGHT EXPOSURE an hour before bed. Use WARM LIGHTING and try AMBER-TINTED GLASSES if screen time is unavoidable.
- **Magnesium Boost:** Add MAGNESIUM-RICH FOODS like SPINACH or PUMPKIN SEEDS to dinner. Magnesium promotes MUSCLE RELAXATION and DEEP SLEEP.
- **Pre-Sleep Rituals:** Take a WARM BATH, sip HERBAL TEA, or practice GUIDED MEDITATION. These signals help the brain SHIFT INTO REST MODE.

Why It Works:

A RESTFUL NIGHT allows the body to REPAIR TISSUES, BALANCE HORMONES, and ENHANCE MEMORY. It also improves WILLPOWER and MOOD STABILITY, which are ESSENTIAL for sticking to new habits.

CREATING A STRESS-RESILIENT ROUTINE

Stress isn't always bad—it can MOTIVATE ACTION—but CHRONIC STRESS disrupts the NERVOUS SYSTEM and WEAKENS IMMUNITY. This week introduces SMALL PRACTICES that BUILD RESILIENCE rather than ELIMINATE STRESS ENTIRELY.

Morning Practices for Calm:

- **Gratitude Journaling (5 Minutes):** Write down THREE THINGS YOU'RE GRATEFUL FOR. This shifts focus from WORRY to ABUNDANCE.
- **Breathwork (3 Minutes):** Practice BOX BREATHING—inhale for FOUR COUNTS, hold for FOUR COUNTS, exhale for FOUR COUNTS, and repeat. This CALMS THE MIND and LOWERS HEART RATE.

Afternoon Stress-Relievers:
- **Nature Breaks (15 Minutes):** Spend time outside, even if it's just a WALK AROUND THE BLOCK. Nature exposure REDUCES CORTISOL and IMPROVES MOOD.
- **Mindful Eating (10 Minutes):** Sit down without distractions and SAVOR EACH BITE. Eating mindfully REDUCES OVEREATING and improves DIGESTION.

Evening Wind-Down Techniques:
- **Aromatherapy:** Diffuse LAVENDER or EUCALYPTUS oil while reading or meditating. Scents trigger the RELAXATION RESPONSE.
- **Reflective Journaling (10 Minutes):** Write about the day's WINS and CHALLENGES. Reflecting builds SELF-AWARENESS and EMOTIONAL CLARITY.

Why It Works:

Resilience isn't about avoiding stress; it's about RECOVERING QUICKLY. These practices RETRAIN THE BRAIN and NERVOUS SYSTEM, making it easier to handle UNEXPECTED PRESSURES.

REINFORCING PROGRESS THROUGH REFLECTION

Reflection is the GLUE that holds new habits together. As Week One unfolds, journaling and tracking progress ENHANCE ACCOUNTABILITY and reveal PATTERNS.

Daily Reflection Prompts:
- WHAT'S ONE THING I DID WELL TODAY?
- WHERE DID I STRUGGLE, AND WHAT CAN I LEARN FROM IT?
- HOW DID MY BODY FEEL BEFORE AND AFTER MEALS OR WORKOUTS?

Why It Works:

Reflection turns TRIAL AND ERROR into PERSONAL INSIGHT. It highlights SMALL WINS and helps you ADJUST STRATEGIES without feeling discouraged.

FINAL THOUGHTS ON WEEK ONE

Week One is about MOMENTUM, not mastery. By focusing on NUTRITION, MOVEMENT, SLEEP, and STRESS MANAGEMENT, you're creating a STRONG FOUNDATION for lasting change. Each small action builds CONFIDENCE and CLARITY, proving that transformation doesn't require PERFECTION—just CONSISTENCY.

5.2 WEEK TWO: ADVANCED STRATEGIES

TAKING GROWTH TO THE NEXT LEVEL

The second week of the 14-DAY TRANSFORMATION PLAN is about EXPANSION. You've already established a SOLID FOUNDATION—now it's time to BUILD UPWARD. This week shifts the focus toward EMOTIONAL WELL-BEING, MENTAL RESILIENCE, and PERSONAL CREATIVITY.

Instead of just managing habits, Week Two encourages you to DEEPEN YOUR PRACTICES and ADAPT THE PLAN to fit your LIFESTYLE and GOALS. The aim isn't to create rigid rules but to develop FLEXIBLE SYSTEMS that empower LONG-TERM GROWTH.

By the end of this week, you'll feel more CONNECTED TO YOURSELF and your PURPOSE. You'll learn how to STRENGTHEN RELATIONSHIPS, reduce MENTAL STRESS, and inject JOY into your routines—all while refining the habits you established during Week One.

EMOTIONAL WELL-BEING: STRENGTHENING RELATIONSHIPS AND REDUCING MENTAL STRESS

Why Emotional Health Matters

EMOTIONAL WELL-BEING is often the INVISIBLE PILLAR of transformation. Without it, even the most disciplined plans can crumble under STRESS, SELF-DOUBT, or EMOTIONAL FATIGUE. This section focuses on nurturing CONNECTION—both with yourself and others—while developing EMOTIONAL TOOLS to REDUCE OVERWHELM.

DEEPENING SELF-CONNECTION
Before focusing on external relationships, it's vital to ANCHOR YOURSELF. Emotional stability begins with SELF-AWARENESS and SELF-COMPASSION.

- **Morning Check-Ins:** Begin each day with 5 MINUTES OF REFLECTION. Ask yourself: WHAT AM I FEELING? and WHAT DO I NEED TODAY? Write down your answers in a JOURNAL to build EMOTIONAL CLARITY.
- **Affirmations That Stick:** Create PERSONAL MANTRAS that reinforce CONFIDENCE and CALM. Phrases like "I AM ENOUGH" or "I RELEASE WHAT I CANNOT CONTROL" act as MENTAL ANCHORS.

STRENGTHENING RELATIONSHIPS
Human connection isn't just emotional—it's BIOLOGICAL. Strong relationships lower STRESS HORMONES and boost HAPPINESS CHEMICALS like OXYTOCIN.

- **Quality Time Over Quantity:** Focus on MEANINGFUL INTERACTIONS. A 10-minute FACE-TO-FACE CONVERSATION with a friend can feel more nourishing than hours of TEXT MESSAGES.
- **Active Listening Practices:** During conversations, practice MIRRORING. Repeat key phrases to show you're FULLY PRESENT and ENGAGED.
- **Express Gratitude Out Loud:** Verbalize appreciation for those around you. Simple statements like "I'M THANKFUL FOR YOUR SUPPORT" deepen bonds and invite RECIPROCITY.

REDUCING MENTAL STRESS
Mental clutter creates EMOTIONAL FOG. Clearing that space allows you to operate with CLARITY and CALM.

- **Mind Dump Technique:** Set aside 10 MINUTES to write down EVERY THOUGHT—no filtering. This technique CLEARS MENTAL NOISE and turns CHAOS INTO CLARITY.
- **Daily Meditation:** Dedicate 5-7 MINUTES to GUIDED BREATHING. Focus on SLOWING THE BREATH and RELAXING TENSION POINTS. Tools like VISUALIZATION can amplify RELAXATION.
- **Boundary Setting Practices:** Practice saying NO with kindness. For example: "I'D LOVE TO HELP, BUT I NEED TO FOCUS ON MY PRIORITIES TODAY." This preserves ENERGY and reduces EMOTIONAL FATIGUE.

INCORPORATING CREATIVITY AND PLAY INTO YOUR ROUTINE
Why Creativity Fuels Transformation
Creativity isn't just about art—it's about PROBLEM-SOLVING, EXPRESSION, and PLAYFULNESS. Engaging in CREATIVE ACTIVITIES rewires the brain, BOOSTS DOPAMINE, and reduces CORTISOL.

DAILY CREATIVE PRACTICES
- **Morning Journaling:** Write STREAM-OF-CONSCIOUSNESS THOUGHTS for 5 MINUTES. Don't edit or censor—just FLOW.
- **Art for Expression:** Spend 10 MINUTES sketching, doodling, or painting. Focus on the PROCESS, not the OUTCOME.
- **Musical Breaks:** Listen to UPLIFTING PLAYLISTS or experiment with INSTRUMENTS. Music stimulates JOY CENTERS in the brain.

INFUSING PLAY INTO DAILY LIFE
Play isn't just for children—it's a STRESS-RELIEF TOOL for adults. Playfulness encourages CURIOSITY, PROBLEM-SOLVING, and EMOTIONAL BALANCE.

- **Outdoor Games:** Toss a frisbee, ride a bike, or play catch. Moving in PLAYFUL WAYS improves MOOD and ENERGY.
- **Game Nights:** Organize GAME NIGHTS with friends or family. Laughter acts as a NATURAL STRESS RELIEVER.
- **Silly Challenges:** Try LIGHT-HEARTED CHALLENGES like balancing a book on your head or dancing to a random song. These moments create JOYFUL MEMORIES.

ADAPTING THE PLAN TO FIT YOUR LIFESTYLE AND GOALS
The Power of Personalization

Transformation isn't ONE-SIZE-FITS-ALL. True change happens when plans are FLEXIBLE enough to accommodate INDIVIDUAL NEEDS. This section focuses on CUSTOMIZING strategies so they align with your PRIORITIES and RHYTHMS.

ASSESSING YOUR NEEDS
- **Daily Reflection Questions:** Ask: WHAT'S WORKING? WHAT'S NOT? Adjust based on these insights.
- **Focus on Priorities:** Highlight ONE OR TWO KEY AREAS—whether it's NUTRITION, STRESS, or MOVEMENT. Avoid SPREADING ENERGY TOO THIN.

PRACTICAL ADJUSTMENTS
- **Time Management:** If mornings feel RUSHED, shift MOVEMENT PRACTICES to lunch breaks or evenings.
- **Food Preferences:** Adapt meals to fit TASTE PREFERENCES—swap PROTEIN SOURCES or VEGETABLE VARIETIES without sacrificing BALANCE.
- **Energy Levels:** Modify workouts based on ENERGY PATTERNS. If you're FATIGUED, swap HIGH-INTENSITY SESSIONS for STRETCHING ROUTINES.

TRACKING PROGRESS WITHOUT PRESSURE
- **Flexible Journaling:** Focus on FEELINGS and SHIFTS IN ENERGY rather than PERFECTION.
- **Weekly Wins List:** Celebrate SMALL VICTORIES—like COOKING A HEALTHY MEAL or GETTING 8 HOURS OF SLEEP.

SUSTAINING GROWTH BEYOND THE TWO WEEKS

The practices from Week Two are designed to CARRY FORWARD. By integrating EMOTIONAL TOOLS, CREATIVE OUTLETS, and PERSONAL FLEXIBILITY, this week empowers you to build RESILIENCE and JOY that last far beyond the transformation plan.

This isn't about finishing a program—it's about BECOMING ADAPTABLE. With the right tools, you'll feel EQUIPPED to handle LIFE'S UNPREDICTABILITY without losing your BALANCE or MOMENTUM.

Conclusion to Chapter 5: The 14-Day Transformation Plan

The 14-DAY TRANSFORMATION PLAN isn't the end of your journey—it's a LAUNCHPAD for continued growth. Over the past two weeks, you've laid the groundwork for SUSTAINABLE HABITS while expanding into EMOTIONAL HEALTH, CREATIVITY, and ADAPTABILITY. By focusing on both STRUCTURE and FLEXIBILITY, this plan has given you the tools to NAVIGATE CHALLENGES without losing MOMENTUM.

As you move forward, CELEBRATE PROGRESS, not perfection. Use what you've learned to PERSONALIZE YOUR ROUTINES and ADJUST AS NEEDED. Growth isn't about RIGID PLANS—it's about RESILIENCE and CONSISTENCY. Whether you continue building on this plan or modify it to fit new goals, remember that LASTING CHANGE happens through INTENTIONAL ACTION and SELF-COMPASSION.

This transformation is YOURS TO SHAPE. Keep leaning into CURIOSITY, JOY, and SELF-CARE—and watch as your efforts unfold into a LIFESTYLE that feels both EMPOWERING and SUSTAINABLE.

CHAPTER 6: DAILY ROUTINES FOR CORTISOL BALANCE

Cortisol, often referred to as the *stress hormone*, plays a central role in regulating energy, metabolism, and the body's response to stress. While it's essential for survival, *chronic imbalances* in cortisol levels can lead to *fatigue, weight gain, anxiety*, and *sleep disturbances*. The good news is that your *daily routines* have the power to influence this hormone—either fueling imbalance or fostering harmony.

This chapter explores *practical strategies* to create daily rhythms that promote *cortisol balance* and restore *inner stability*. By incorporating *intentional habits* into your mornings, afternoons, and evenings, you can shift from cycles of *overwhelm* to states of *calm and focus*. Whether it's starting your day with *breathing exercises* to ground your mind, *nutrient-dense meals* to fuel your energy, or *relaxation techniques* to prepare for restful sleep, every small choice contributes to *lasting transformation*.

Balancing cortisol isn't about *rigid schedules* or *perfection*. It's about *consistent rituals* that fit into *your lifestyle* and evolve with your needs. This chapter equips you with tools to *lower stress, build resilience*, and create habits that are *sustainable*—not just for days, but for *a lifetime*.

6.1 CRAFTING YOUR MORNING ROUTINE

The morning sets the tone for the entire day. How you start determines how your BODY, MIND, and NERVOUS SYSTEM respond to stressors, challenges, and opportunities. Crafting a DELIBERATE MORNING ROUTINE helps regulate CORTISOL LEVELS, preventing spikes that lead to fatigue, irritability, and brain fog. This section explores PRACTICAL STEPS to create mornings that ENERGIZE without overwhelming, blending CALMNESS and FOCUS for an INTENTIONAL START.

THE IMPORTANCE OF A GROUNDED MORNING

Mornings are when CORTISOL PRODUCTION NATURALLY PEAKS. Known as the CORTISOL AWAKENING RESPONSE, this surge is designed to BOOST ALERTNESS and PREPARE THE BODY FOR ACTION. However, modern lifestyles—characterized by RUSHED SCHEDULES, TECHNOLOGY OVERLOAD, and SKIPPED BREAKFASTS—often cause cortisol to OVERREACT, flooding the body with STRESS SIGNALS.

A GROUNDED MORNING ROUTINE helps SMOOTH CORTISOL FLUCTUATIONS, promoting STABILITY rather than SPIKES. It encourages the PARASYMPATHETIC NERVOUS SYSTEM—responsible for REST AND DIGESTION—to stay ACTIVE and prevents the FIGHT-OR-FLIGHT RESPONSE from dominating.

STEP 1: BREATHING EXERCISES TO START THE DAY

Before reaching for your phone or diving into tasks, pause. A few minutes of DEEP, INTENTIONAL BREATHING immediately calms the NERVOUS SYSTEM, signaling safety and grounding the body.

Breathwork Technique: Box Breathing

- HOW TO PRACTICE: Inhale through the nose for FOUR COUNTS. Hold the breath for FOUR COUNTS. Exhale slowly for FOUR COUNTS. Hold again for FOUR COUNTS. Repeat for FIVE ROUNDS.
- WHY IT WORKS: Box breathing activates the VAGUS NERVE, reducing SYMPATHETIC AROUSAL (the stress response) and LOWERING CORTISOL LEVELS.

Alternative Method: 4-7-8 Breathing

- HOW TO PRACTICE: Inhale deeply through the nose for FOUR COUNTS. Hold for SEVEN COUNTS. Exhale fully through the mouth for EIGHT COUNTS. Repeat for FOUR ROUNDS.
- WHY IT WORKS: This technique promotes OXYGEN FLOW, RELAXES MUSCLES, and enhances FOCUS by LOWERING HEART RATE.

STEP 2: JOURNALING FOR MENTAL CLARITY
After breathing, transition into journaling. Writing down THOUGHTS, INTENTIONS, and GRATITUDE acts as a mental DECLUTTERING TOOL. It prevents OVERTHINKING and reduces MORNING ANXIETY.

Morning Journaling Prompts:
- WHAT AM I GRATEFUL FOR TODAY?
- WHAT'S ONE POSITIVE INTENTION I CAN SET FOR THE DAY?
- WHAT'S THE BIGGEST PRIORITY I WANT TO FOCUS ON?

Why Journaling Works:

Journaling shifts attention from WORRY to CLARITY. It engages the PREFRONTAL CORTEX—responsible for DECISION-MAKING—and decreases activity in the AMYGDALA, which controls FEAR RESPONSES.

STEP 3: ENERGIZING YET STRESS-FREE BREAKFAST OPTIONS
A cortisol-friendly breakfast fuels the body without causing blood sugar spikes. Instead of HIGH-CARB or SUGAR-LADEN MEALS, opt for PROTEIN-RICH, HEALTHY-FAT-BASED options that STABILIZE ENERGY.

Balanced Breakfast Ideas:
1. AVOCADO TOAST WITH POACHED EGGS – Provides PROTEIN and MONOUNSATURATED FATS to keep you SATIATED longer.
2. GREEK YOGURT WITH BERRIES AND CHIA SEEDS – Rich in PROBIOTICS, FIBER, and OMEGA-3S to SUPPORT DIGESTION and REDUCE INFLAMMATION.
3. SMOOTHIE BOWL WITH SPINACH, BANANA, ALMOND BUTTER, AND HEMP SEEDS – Delivers MAGNESIUM, POTASSIUM, and HEALTHY FATS for NERVOUS SYSTEM SUPPORT.
4. OATMEAL WITH NUT BUTTER, CINNAMON, AND WALNUTS – A mix of COMPLEX CARBS and PROTEIN that BALANCES BLOOD SUGAR.

The Science Behind Breakfast Choices:
- PROTEIN helps REGULATE DOPAMINE, keeping you FOCUSED.
- HEALTHY FATS slow GLUCOSE ABSORPTION, preventing ENERGY CRASHES.
- FIBER supports GUT HEALTH, which influences MOOD REGULATION.

STEP 4: SUNLIGHT AND MOVEMENT FOR CORTISOL REGULATION
After breakfast, step outside or move your body gently. Sunlight exposure within 30 MINUTES of waking helps SYNCHRONIZE CIRCADIAN RHYTHMS and stabilizes MORNING CORTISOL.

Morning Walk or Stretch Routine:
- Take a 10-MINUTE WALK outdoors, focusing on BREATHING DEEPLY and NOTICING SURROUNDINGS.
- Follow with DYNAMIC STRETCHES like CAT-COW POSES, FORWARD BENDS, and SIDE LUNGES to STIMULATE CIRCULATION.

Why Movement Matters:

Physical activity promotes ENDORPHIN RELEASE—the brain's NATURAL STRESS RELIEVER—and reduces CORTISOL BUILDUP. Combining movement with NATURE EXPOSURE magnifies the effects by activating DOPAMINE RECEPTORS linked to HAPPINESS.

STEP 5: MORNING RITUALS TO LIMIT TECHNOLOGY STRESS
Resist the urge to check your phone first thing. Screens—especially emails, notifications, and social media—trigger a DOPAMINE LOOP, increasing MENTAL CLUTTER.

Create a No-Phone Zone:
- Dedicate the FIRST HOUR of the day to being OFFLINE.
- Replace phone-checking habits with MUSIC, PODCASTS, or INSPIRATIONAL READINGS.

Why It Works:

Minimizing EARLY-MORNING STIMULI reduces COGNITIVE OVERLOAD and prevents STRESS HORMONES from spiking unnecessarily.

STEP 6: HYDRATION FOR HORMONAL BALANCE

Hydrate before caffeine. Overnight, the body becomes DEHYDRATED, which can amplify STRESS RESPONSES. Start your day with WARM LEMON WATER or HERBAL TEAS.

Hydration Recipes for Cortisol Control:

1. WARM LEMON AND GINGER WATER – Stimulates DIGESTION and reduces INFLAMMATION.
2. CUCUMBER AND MINT INFUSED WATER – Provides ELECTROLYTES for NERVOUS SYSTEM STABILITY.
3. GREEN TEA WITH LEMON – Rich in L-THEANINE, which CALMS THE MIND.

Why Hydration Matters:

Dehydration elevates CORTISOL, increases FATIGUE, and disrupts FOCUS. Drinking water before caffeine keeps HORMONAL RHYTHMS steady.

STEP 7: SETTING INTENTIONS AND AFFIRMATIONS

Before stepping into your day, set an intention. This isn't about creating a TO-DO LIST. It's about focusing your ENERGY and MINDSET.

Daily Affirmations:

- "I AM GROUNDED, CALM, AND PREPARED FOR THE DAY AHEAD."
- "I RELEASE STRESS AND EMBRACE CLARITY."
- "I AM IN CONTROL OF MY THOUGHTS AND ENERGY."

Why Intentions Work:

Intentional thinking REWIRES NEURAL PATHWAYS, training the brain to ANTICIPATE CALMNESS instead of REACTING TO STRESS.

CLOSING MORNING ROUTINE THOUGHTS

Morning routines are less about PERFECTION and more about CONSISTENCY. Small, intentional steps—like BREATHWORK, JOURNALING, and PROTEIN-RICH BREAKFASTS—signal to your body that it's SAFE and SUPPORTED. As cortisol stabilizes, you'll notice BETTER FOCUS, IMPROVED MOOD, and a MORE BALANCED START. Craft mornings that work WITH YOUR BIOLOGY, and let them become the ANCHOR for your daily rhythm.

6.2 MIDDAY STRATEGIES FOR ENERGY AND FOCUS

Maintaining CONSISTENT ENERGY LEVELS and MENTAL CLARITY throughout the day is essential for regulating CORTISOL BALANCE. The midday hours can be a TURNING POINT—either a time to REINVIGORATE your body and mind or a period where SLUGGISHNESS and STRESS take over. Developing INTENTIONAL STRATEGIES during this window can prevent ENERGY CRASHES, IRRITABILITY, and the SPIKES in CORTISOL that often occur when blood sugar and focus fluctuate.

This section delves into PRACTICAL MIDDAY HABITS that promote STABILITY and SUSTAINED PERFORMANCE. From BALANCED MEALS that prevent BLOOD SUGAR SWINGS to MINDFUL BREATHING TECHNIQUES that RESET MENTAL FOCUS, these strategies are designed to help you stay CENTERED and ENERGIZED. You'll also learn how MOVEMENT, HYDRATION, and RESTORATIVE PAUSES can create MOMENTUM rather than FATIGUE as the day progresses.

AVOIDING BLOOD SUGAR SPIKES AND MIDDAY SLUMPS

Understanding the Cortisol-Blood Sugar Connection

Cortisol plays a DIRECT ROLE in BLOOD SUGAR REGULATION. It triggers the release of GLUCOSE into the bloodstream during STRESSFUL SITUATIONS, ensuring the body has enough ENERGY to respond. However, IMBALANCES in blood sugar—caused by skipping meals, consuming HIGH-GLYCEMIC FOODS, or overeating—can cause SHARP SPIKES and CRASHES. These fluctuations often lead to FATIGUE, BRAIN FOG, and IRRITABILITY, signaling the body to release even more CORTISOL.

The goal is to STABILIZE BLOOD SUGAR LEVELS through NUTRIENT-DENSE FOODS and BALANCED MACRONUTRIENTS. This approach prevents the ROLLERCOASTER EFFECT that taxes your ADRENAL GLANDS and contributes to CORTISOL DYSREGULATION.

Crafting a Cortisol-Friendly Lunch

A BALANCED LUNCH should include:

- HIGH-QUALITY PROTEIN (grilled chicken, salmon, lentils) to sustain ENERGY and MUSCLE REPAIR.
- HEALTHY FATS (avocado, nuts, olive oil) to SLOW DIGESTION and provide SATIETY.
- COMPLEX CARBOHYDRATES (quinoa, sweet potatoes, leafy greens) to supply STEADY GLUCOSE RELEASE.
- FIBER-RICH VEGETABLES (broccoli, spinach, zucchini) to support DIGESTION and GUT HEALTH.

Example: A GRAIN BOWL with QUINOA, ROASTED VEGETABLES, CHICKPEAS, AVOCADO SLICES, and a drizzle of TAHINI DRESSING delivers a STEADY RELEASE OF ENERGY without overwhelming your DIGESTIVE SYSTEM.

Timing and Portion Control

Eating TOO LITTLE or TOO MUCH can strain CORTISOL REGULATION. Portion control keeps HUNGER HORMONES like GHRELIN in check, preventing OVEREATING later in the day. Aiming to eat within THREE TO FOUR HOURS of breakfast ensures BLOOD SUGAR STABILITY and prevents AFTERNOON CRAVINGS.

Smart Snacks for Sustained Energy

Keep PORTABLE SNACKS on hand to avoid ENERGY CRASHES. Look for combinations of PROTEIN and HEALTHY FATS such as:

- HARD-BOILED EGGS with HUMMUS.
- NUT BUTTER on APPLE SLICES.
- GREEK YOGURT topped with CHIA SEEDS.
- TRAIL MIX with ALMONDS and DRIED BERRIES.

These snacks PREVENT CORTISOL SPIKES while maintaining STEADY GLUCOSE LEVELS.

QUICK MINDFULNESS BREAKS TO RESET MENTAL FOCUS

The Power of Intentional Pauses

Modern schedules often leave little room for MENTAL REST, causing COGNITIVE FATIGUE and HEIGHTENED CORTISOL LEVELS. Taking SHORT, MINDFUL BREAKS allows your NERVOUS SYSTEM to shift from a STRESS RESPONSE to a STATE OF RELAXATION. These MICRO-RECOVERIES improve MENTAL CLARITY and PRODUCTIVITY.

Breathwork for Instant Calm

Controlled breathing resets the PARASYMPATHETIC NERVOUS SYSTEM, signaling SAFETY and CALM. Try the 4-7-8 BREATHING TECHNIQUE:

- INHALE through the nose for FOUR SECONDS.
- HOLD the breath for SEVEN SECONDS.
- EXHALE slowly through the mouth for EIGHT SECONDS.

Repeat this cycle FOUR TIMES during breaks to RELEASE TENSION.

Progressive Muscle Relaxation

Progressive muscle relaxation (PMR) reduces PHYSICAL TENSION by focusing on SPECIFIC MUSCLE GROUPS. Start by TENSING a muscle group (like your SHOULDERS) for FIVE SECONDS, then RELEASE and focus on the RELAXATION SENSATION. Work through the BODY from HEAD TO TOE.

Visualization Techniques

Guided imagery can INTERRUPT STRESS PATTERNS by creating a MENTAL ESCAPE. Picture yourself in a PEACEFUL ENVIRONMENT—a FOREST TRAIL or CALM BEACH. Engage all FIVE SENSES in your visualization to ANCHOR YOURSELF in CALMNESS.

The 10-Minute Rule

Set aside 10 MINUTES midday for SELF-CHECK-INS. Use this time to JOURNAL quick thoughts, STRETCH, or listen to SOOTHING MUSIC. These brief rituals GROUND YOUR EMOTIONS and SHARPEN FOCUS.

STRETCHING AND MOVEMENT FOR ENERGY AND CIRCULATION

Breaking Sedentary Patterns

Long hours at a desk can cause MUSCLE STIFFNESS and REDUCED CIRCULATION, leading to MENTAL FATIGUE. Incorporating MOVEMENT into your midday routine releases ENDORPHINS and lowers CORTISOL.

Dynamic Stretching

Focus on DYNAMIC STRETCHES that STIMULATE BLOOD FLOW:

- NECK ROLLS to EASE TENSION in the SHOULDERS.
- TORSO TWISTS to IMPROVE MOBILITY.
- HAMSTRING STRETCHES to REDUCE STIFFNESS.
- ARM CIRCLES to LOOSEN JOINTS.

Perform TWO TO THREE MINUTES of stretching every HOUR.

Desk-Friendly Exercises

Incorporate movements that REQUIRE MINIMAL SPACE:

- SEATED LEG LIFTS.
- STANDING CALF RAISES.
- CHAIR SQUATS.

These activities prevent CIRCULATION ISSUES and boost ENERGY FLOW.

Walking Breaks

Taking a 10- TO 15-MINUTE WALK outdoors during lunch provides NATURAL SUNLIGHT, which regulates your CIRCADIAN RHYTHM and CORTISOL LEVELS. Exposure to FRESH AIR also stimulates SEROTONIN PRODUCTION, improving MOOD.

HYDRATION FOR CORTISOL REGULATION

The Role of Water in Stress Response

Dehydration triggers the release of CORTISOL, amplifying STRESS. Proper HYDRATION supports ADRENAL FUNCTION and maintains ELECTROLYTE BALANCE.

Optimal Water Intake

Aim for at least HALF YOUR BODY WEIGHT in OUNCES OF WATER daily. Add LEMON SLICES or HERBAL INFUSIONS for flavor and ANTIOXIDANTS.

Hydrating Foods

Include WATER-RICH FOODS like CUCUMBERS, MELONS, CELERY, and ORANGES to boost HYDRATION LEVELS.

SUSTAINING ENERGY WITHOUT STIMULANTS

Limiting Caffeine Intake

While COFFEE and ENERGY DRINKS may seem like a quick fix, they often SPIKE CORTISOL and lead to CRASHES. Replace AFTERNOON CAFFEINE with GREEN TEA, which provides L-THEANINE for CALM FOCUS.

Adaptogenic Teas

Herbal teas like ASHWAGANDHA or HOLY BASIL support ADRENAL HEALTH and STRESS RESILIENCE.

Midday strategies are not about FIXING FATIGUE but BUILDING RESILIENCE. Whether through BALANCED NUTRITION, MINDFUL BREAKS, or STRETCHING, these tools sustain ENERGY and MENTAL CLARITY. Over time, they create HABITS that allow you to STAY CALM and FOCUSED even during life's MOST DEMANDING MOMENTS.

6.3 EVENING RELAXATION TECHNIQUES

The evening hours hold TRANSFORMATIVE POWER. They set the stage for DEEP REST, PHYSICAL RECOVERY, and EMOTIONAL BALANCE. Yet, for many, evenings feel RUSHED, OVERSTIMULATING, or UNSETTLED. Emails linger, screens glow, and worries brew. These habits keep CORTISOL LEVELS ELEVATED well into the night, disrupting the NATURAL RHYTHM needed for quality sleep.

By embracing EVENING RITUALS, you can SHIFT YOUR BODY out of a STRESS-DRIVEN STATE and into CALM READINESS FOR REST. This section introduces INTENTIONAL TECHNIQUES—from AROMATHERAPY to PRE-BEDTIME ROUTINES—designed to SIGNAL SAFETY, LOWER CORTISOL, and prepare both MIND AND BODY for the restorative sleep they crave.

UNWINDING WITH AROMATHERAPY AND WARM BATHS

Scent and sensation deeply influence relaxation. Aromatherapy taps into the LIMBIC SYSTEM—the brain's EMOTIONAL CENTER—triggering SOOTHING RESPONSES. When paired with a WARM BATH, this combination amplifies RELAXATION by promoting MUSCLE RELEASE and IMPROVED CIRCULATION.

Essential Oils for Evening Calm:

- LAVENDER – Known for its CALMING AND SEDATIVE EFFECTS. Studies suggest it reduces HEART RATE and BLOOD PRESSURE.
- CHAMOMILE – Eases NERVOUS TENSION and supports MENTAL CLARITY.
- FRANKINCENSE – Grounds the MIND and deepens BREATHING.
- YLANG-YLANG – Lowers STRESS LEVELS and promotes a sense of COMFORT.

Bath Ritual for Stress Relief:

1. Fill the tub with WARM WATER, ensuring it's COMFORTABLY HEATED but not overly hot.
2. Add EPSOM SALTS (rich in MAGNESIUM) to relax MUSCLES.
3. Mix 10 DROPS of essential oil with a CARRIER OIL (like COCONUT OIL) before dispersing it into the water.
4. Dim the lights and use CANDLES or SOFT MUSIC to create a CALMING ATMOSPHERE.

No Bathtub? No Problem:

For those without a tub, a WARM SHOWER with essential oils or a FOOT SOAK in scented water can mimic the effects of a FULL-BODY SOAK.

BREATHWORK AND MEDITATION FOR NERVOUS SYSTEM RESET

Evenings often carry MENTAL RESIDUE from the day—unfinished tasks, emails, or deadlines. Breathwork and meditation act as ANCHORS, pulling the mind into the PRESENT and RESETTING THE NERVOUS SYSTEM.

Breathing Patterns for Cortisol Control:

- BOX BREATHING – Inhale for 4 COUNTS, hold for 4 COUNTS, exhale for 4 COUNTS, and pause for 4 COUNTS. Repeat 5-7 CYCLES.
- ALTERNATE NOSTRIL BREATHING – Clears MENTAL CLUTTER and balances BRAIN HEMISPHERES.
- EXTENDED EXHALE TECHNIQUE – Emphasizes LONG EXHALES to signal PARASYMPATHETIC ACTIVATION.

Guided Meditations Before Bed:
- Body Scan Meditation – Focuses on RELEASING TENSION from each body part.
- Loving-Kindness Meditation – Encourages POSITIVE EMOTIONS to counteract WORRY LOOPS.
- Visualization Practices – Imagine CALM SCENES like beaches, forests, or lakes.

CALMING ACTIVITIES THAT PROMOTE STILLNESS

Sometimes the mind resists stillness. In these moments, GENTLE ACTIVITIES can act as STEPPING STONES to deeper relaxation.

Evening Ritual Ideas:
- JOURNALING GRATITUDE – Reflecting on SMALL WINS fosters a sense of COMPLETION.
- PUZZLES OR COLORING – Engages the CREATIVE BRAIN and redirects ANXIOUS ENERGY.
- READING FICTION OR POETRY – Avoids the MENTAL STIMULATION caused by NON-FICTION.
- KNITTING OR DRAWING – Uses REPETITIVE MOTIONS to create CALM FOCUS.

Avoid Stimulants After 6 p.m.:

Cutting CAFFEINE and SUGAR in the evening prevents CORTISOL SPIKES. Opt for HERBAL TEAS like PEPPERMINT or LEMON BALM.

PRE-BEDTIME RITUALS FOR BETTER SLEEP

The HOUR BEFORE BED is a TRANSITION ZONE. Treat it like PREPARING FOR TAKEOFF. Just as planes need WIND-DOWN PROCEDURES, your body craves PREDICTABLE SIGNALS to POWER DOWN.

Key Rituals to Establish Sleep Readiness:
- DIM THE LIGHTS EARLY – Lowering light exposure triggers MELATONIN RELEASE. Use WARM-TONED BULBS or SALT LAMPS.
- TECH DETOX – Shut off SCREENS at least 30 MINUTES before bed. The BLUE LIGHT emitted suppresses MELATONIN.
- STRETCH AND UNWIND – Gentle YOGA POSES like CHILD'S POSE or LEGS-UP-THE-WALL release MUSCLE TENSION.
- WEIGHTED BLANKETS – Provide DEEP PRESSURE STIMULATION, which reduces CORTISOL.
- SLEEP JOURNALS – Write down WORRIES or THOUGHTS to CLEAR MENTAL CLUTTER.

Herbal Support for Sleep Enhancement:
- MAGNESIUM GLYCINATE – Calms NERVOUS TENSION and improves SLEEP QUALITY.
- ASHWAGANDHA – An ADAPTOGEN that lowers STRESS HORMONES.
- VALERIAN ROOT – Known for its MILD SEDATIVE PROPERTIES.

SOUND THERAPY AND NATURE SOUNDS FOR DEEPER SLEEP

The right SOUNDSCAPE can guide your brain into RESTORATIVE STATES. Low-frequency sounds and BINAURAL BEATS mimic MEDITATIVE RHYTHMS.

Recommended Sounds:
- RAINFALL OR OCEAN WAVES – Mimics NATURAL RHYTHMS.
- WHITE NOISE MACHINES – Masks BACKGROUND DISTRACTIONS.
- 432 HZ MUSIC – Known for CALMING EFFECTS.

CREATING A CONSISTENT SLEEP SCHEDULE
Consistency reinforces CIRCADIAN RHYTHMS. Aim to go to bed and wake up at the SAME TIME DAILY, even on weekends. This anchors your BODY CLOCK, lowering CORTISOL VARIABILITY.

Sleep Hygiene Checklist:
- Keep the bedroom COOL (around 65°F).
- Invest in BLACKOUT CURTAINS or SLEEP MASKS.
- Avoid HEAVY MEALS within TWO HOURS of bedtime.
- Use AROMATHERAPY DIFFUSERS overnight.

FINAL TOUCHPOINTS FOR EVENING CALM
Evenings should signal a GENTLE DECELERATION. Whether it's a CUP OF CHAMOMILE TEA, a GUIDED MEDITATION, or a WARM BATH, the focus remains on INTENTIONAL CALM.

When the BODY FEELS SAFE, it allows cortisol to DROP NATURALLY. Evening routines aren't about RIGIDITY; they're about TRUSTING THE PROCESS. Each ritual REINFORCES SAFETY, helping the nervous system to RELEASE TENSION and embrace RESTORATIVE SLEEP.

6.4 MAKING HABITS STICK FOR THE LONG TERM
Creating daily routines that support CORTISOL BALANCE is more than a temporary fix—it's a commitment to LASTING CHANGE. Many people start strong, but consistency often fades when MOTIVATION DIPS, LIFE GETS BUSY, or UNEXPECTED CHALLENGES ARISE. The good news is that SUSTAINABLE HABITS aren't built on WILLPOWER ALONE. They rely on STRATEGIC FRAMEWORKS, EMOTIONAL ALIGNMENT, and PRACTICAL TOOLS that make following through EASIER, NOT HARDER.

This section focuses on BUILDING SYSTEMS that keep habits INTACT, even when circumstances shift. It also explores how to NAVIGATE SETBACKS without derailing progress. True transformation happens when routines stop feeling like CHORES and start becoming part of your IDENTITY.

TIPS FOR BUILDING CONSISTENT AND SUSTAINABLE ROUTINES
1. Anchor New Habits to Existing Routines
The easiest way to CEMENT A HABIT is to tie it to something you already do. This is called HABIT STACKING, and it eliminates the need to REMEMBER or FORCE new actions.

- Example: Pair MORNING BREATHING EXERCISES with brushing your teeth.
- Example: Journal for 5 MINUTES right after making your morning coffee.
- Example: Meditate immediately after TURNING OFF YOUR WORK LAPTOP at the end of the day.

Attaching new habits to CONSISTENT TRIGGERS reduces DECISION FATIGUE and makes following through AUTOMATIC.

2. Start Small and Build Gradually
Big changes often fail because they feel OVERWHELMING. Instead of aiming for a COMPLETE OVERHAUL, focus on TINY WINS.

- Begin with 2 MINUTES of mindfulness before bed instead of 20 MINUTES.
- Swap ONE HIGH-SUGAR SNACK for a PROTEIN-RICH OPTION instead of revamping your entire diet.
- Commit to stretching for just 5 MINUTES rather than an entire yoga flow.

Small wins COMPOUND OVER TIME. Once habits feel EFFORTLESS, you can EXPAND them naturally.

3. Use Visual Cues to Reinforce Behavior

Environmental design plays a HUGE ROLE in sustaining habits. Making DESIRED ACTIONS OBVIOUS and ACCESSIBLE reduces FRICTION.

- Keep a GRATITUDE JOURNAL on your nightstand as a reminder to write.
- Place a YOGA MAT in a visible spot instead of hiding it in the closet.
- Set up a DIFFUSER near your bed to encourage nightly aromatherapy.

OUT OF SIGHT, OUT OF MIND applies to habits. Keep your tools VISIBLE and READY TO USE.

4. Reward Progress, Not Perfection

Many routines fall apart because people feel discouraged when they MISS A DAY. Instead of chasing PERFECTION, focus on CONSISTENCY OVER TIME.

- Celebrate SMALL VICTORIES like completing 3 DAYS IN A ROW of mindfulness exercises.
- Track progress visually with a HABIT TRACKER or CALENDAR MARKS.
- Reward yourself with NON-FOOD TREATS, such as a SPA NIGHT or NEW BOOK, after hitting a WEEKLY GOAL.

Consistency is STRENGTHENED BY CELEBRATION. Progress—even if IMPERFECT—builds MOMENTUM.

5. Set Specific, Measurable Goals

Vague intentions like "I WANT TO BE LESS STRESSED" lack the CLARITY needed for action. Instead, break goals into MEASURABLE STEPS.

- "Practice 5 MINUTES of breathwork before bed, 5 DAYS A WEEK."
- "Replace my MIDDAY COFFEE with GREEN TEA for 2 WEEKS."
- "Write in my journal 3 NIGHTS this week."

Clear goals make it easier to TRACK PROGRESS and COURSE-CORRECT.

HOW TO HANDLE SETBACKS

Even the MOST COMMITTED ROUTINES face obstacles. Illness, travel, deadlines, and emotional stress can DERAIL HABITS. What matters most is how you RESPOND.

1. Reframe Setbacks as Temporary, Not Permanent

Missed routines don't erase progress. Instead of SELF-CRITICISM, remind yourself that ONE OFF DAY won't undo WEEKS OF EFFORT. Use setbacks as LEARNING MOMENTS.

- "WHAT CAUSED ME TO SKIP MY HABIT?"
- "HOW CAN I MAKE IT EASIER NEXT TIME?"

Self-compassion keeps you MOTIVATED and helps you BOUNCE BACK.

2. Prepare for Obstacles in Advance

Proactive planning makes setbacks LESS DISRUPTIVE.

- Traveling? Pack TRAVEL-SIZED ESSENTIAL OILS and a JOURNAL.
- Tight schedule? Shorten the routine (e.g., 2-MINUTE MEDITATION).
- Low energy? Swap a BATH for a FOOT SOAK or use AROMATHERAPY SPRAY.

Anticipating challenges removes the ALL-OR-NOTHING MINDSET.

3. Focus on Identity Over Goals

Lasting change happens when routines feel like EXPRESSIONS OF WHO YOU ARE. Instead of saying, "I WANT TO MANAGE STRESS," tell yourself, "I'M SOMEONE WHO PRIORITIZES CALM AND BALANCE."

Identity-based habits are INTRINSIC, making them HARDER TO BREAK.

PRACTICAL TOOLS FOR LONG-TERM SUCCESS

1. Journals and Trackers
Writing reinforces ACCOUNTABILITY. Use trackers to measure habits or write END-OF-DAY REFLECTIONS.

2. Accountability Partners
Partnering with a friend can add SUPPORT and MOTIVATION. Sharing goals creates EXTERNAL ACCOUNTABILITY.

3. Apps and Reminders
Apps like CALM or HEADSPACE send GENTLE REMINDERS to practice mindfulness or breathwork. Use PHONE ALARMS to signal breaks.

4. Visual Habit Prompts
Sticky notes with affirmations like "PAUSE AND BREATHE" or "5 MINUTES FOR ME" remind you to PAUSE during busy days.

BUILDING A RESILIENT MINDSET

A FLEXIBLE MINDSET makes habits SUSTAINABLE. Stressful periods don't have to derail progress—they can deepen SELF-AWARENESS.

- Learn to PIVOT, not QUIT.
- Focus on PROGRESS OVER PERFECTION.
- Celebrate the PROCESS, not just the OUTCOME.

FINAL THOUGHTS ON LONG-TERM CHANGE

Building habits that balance CORTISOL LEVELS isn't about QUICK FIXES. It's about creating RITUALS that feel NOURISHING rather than RESTRICTIVE. When routines reflect your VALUES, they become ANCHORS—steadying you in moments of UNCERTAINTY and helping you return to CALM.

By crafting INTENTIONAL PRACTICES, celebrating SMALL WINS, and navigating SETBACKS WITH GRACE, you create a foundation that supports LASTING TRANSFORMATION.

Conclusion to Chapter 6: Daily Routines for Cortisol Balance

Balancing CORTISOL LEVELS isn't about QUICK FIXES or TEMPORARY DETOXES. It's about RETHINKING YOUR DAILY PATTERNS to align with your body's NATURAL RHYTHMS. The routines explored in this chapter—whether MORNING BREATHING EXERCISES, MIDDAY MINDFULNESS BREAKS, or EVENING RELAXATION RITUALS—are designed to help you RESET, REFOCUS, and RECHARGE.

When these habits become SECOND NATURE, they don't just REDUCE STRESS—they lay the foundation for LASTING WELL-BEING. Small, CONSISTENT ACTIONS create a CUMULATIVE EFFECT, rewiring your NERVOUS SYSTEM and HORMONAL PATTERNS for BETTER HEALTH.

True transformation doesn't happen overnight. It grows through PRACTICE, PATIENCE, and SELF-COMPASSION. By making CORTISOL-CONSCIOUS ROUTINES a part of your lifestyle, you build not just BALANCE, but a RESILIENT MINDSET—ready to handle life's CHALLENGES with CALM AND CLARITY.

CHAPTER 7: NATURAL SUPPORT FOR STRESS REDUCTION

In today's fast-paced world, stress has become a near-constant companion, often leaving us feeling EXHAUSTED, UNFOCUSED, and OVERWHELMED. While occasional stress is a natural part of life, CHRONIC STRESS can throw the body's delicate hormonal balance into disarray, leading to FATIGUE, ANXIETY, and BURNOUT. The good news is that nature offers a treasure trove of remedies that can help RESTORE CALM, REBALANCE CORTISOL LEVELS, and SUPPORT OVERALL WELL-BEING.

This chapter dives into the HEALING POWER of NATURAL TOOLS designed to combat stress—focusing on HERBS, SUPPLEMENTS, ESSENTIAL OILS, and DIY REMEDIES. Whether it's the ADAPTOGENIC PROPERTIES of ASHWAGANDHA and RHODIOLA, the MAGNESIUM-RICH SUPPLEMENTS that promote RELAXATION, or the SOOTHING AROMAS of LAVENDER and CHAMOMILE, these resources work with the body's natural systems to REDUCE TENSION and ENHANCE RESILIENCE.

From NOURISHING TEAS and AROMATIC BATHS to TARGETED SUPPLEMENTS and CUSTOM BLENDS, the strategies outlined here emphasize SIMPLE, EFFECTIVE PRACTICES you can incorporate into daily life. By tapping into nature's pharmacy, you can create PERSONALIZED ROUTINES that promote CALMNESS, CLARITY, and INNER STRENGTH—empowering you to face challenges with GRACE and CONFIDENCE.

7.1 HERBS AND ADAPTOGENS FOR CORTISOL BALANCE

The natural world offers a powerful toolkit for restoring BALANCE and RESILIENCE in the face of STRESS. Herbs and adaptogens—plants with unique properties that help the body ADAPT TO STRESSORS—can be GAME-CHANGERS for those seeking to support CORTISOL REGULATION naturally. Unlike synthetic solutions, these botanicals often work SYNERGISTICALLY with the body, enhancing ENERGY, FOCUS, and CALM without causing DEPENDENCY or SIDE EFFECTS.

Adaptogens are celebrated for their ability to MODULATE CORTISOL LEVELS, whether they are TOO HIGH due to ACUTE STRESS or TOO LOW as a result of CHRONIC FATIGUE. By targeting the HYPOTHALAMIC-PITUITARY-ADRENAL (HPA) AXIS, these herbs assist in BALANCING HORMONES and RESTORING EQUILIBRIUM.

This section explores the most EFFECTIVE ADAPTOGENS and herbs for CORTISOL BALANCE, highlighting their BENEFITS, MECHANISMS OF ACTION, and SAFE USAGE GUIDELINES.

ASHWAGANDHA: THE ROOT OF CALM RESILIENCE

Key Benefits

Ashwagandha (WITHANIA SOMNIFERA), a staple in AYURVEDIC MEDICINE, is renowned for its ability to LOWER CORTISOL LEVELS and SOOTHE ANXIETY. This root acts as a TONIC for the ADRENAL GLANDS, nourishing the body's ability to handle PHYSICAL and EMOTIONAL STRESS.

Studies indicate that DAILY SUPPLEMENTATION with ashwagandha may reduce MORNING CORTISOL by up to 30%, leading to IMPROVED MOOD, ENHANCED FOCUS, and BETTER SLEEP QUALITY.

How It Works

Ashwagandha influences the HPA AXIS by regulating CORTICOTROPIN-RELEASING HORMONE (CRH), which initiates the STRESS RESPONSE. Its bioactive compounds, called WITHANOLIDES, have been shown to:

- REDUCE INFLAMMATION.
- ENHANCE GABA ACTIVITY in the brain for a CALMING EFFECT.
- STABILIZE BLOOD SUGAR, preventing SPIKES that trigger CORTISOL RELEASE.

Safe Usage

- DOSAGE: Typically 300–600 MG per day of a STANDARDIZED EXTRACT.
- TIMING: Best taken in the EVENING to promote RELAXATION and support SLEEP.
- PRECAUTIONS: Avoid during PREGNANCY or if using THYROID MEDICATIONS, as it may influence HORMONAL LEVELS.

RHODIOLA ROSEA: THE ENERGY RESTORER
Key Benefits
Rhodiola rosea is prized for its ability to ENHANCE STAMINA and MENTAL CLARITY while simultaneously LOWERING CORTISOL. Often referred to as the ARCTIC ROOT, it's ideal for those experiencing MENTAL FATIGUE or feeling OVERWHELMED.

Clinical trials show that Rhodiola can:

- REDUCE CORTISOL SPIKES during STRESSFUL EVENTS.
- INCREASE SEROTONIN and DOPAMINE production, improving MOOD.
- BOOST PHYSICAL ENDURANCE and COGNITIVE PERFORMANCE.

How It Works
Rhodiola's active compounds, ROSAVINS and SALIDROSIDE, regulate CORTISOL SECRETION by modulating the SYMPATHETIC NERVOUS SYSTEM. They also act as ANTIOXIDANTS, protecting the body from OXIDATIVE STRESS caused by CHRONIC CORTISOL ELEVATION.

Safe Usage
- DOSAGE: 200–600 MG per day, depending on CONCENTRATION.
- TIMING: Best taken in the MORNING or EARLY AFTERNOON to avoid DISRUPTING SLEEP.
- PRECAUTIONS: May cause MILD JITTERINESS in SENSITIVE INDIVIDUALS. Start with a LOWER DOSE and increase gradually.

GINSENG: THE ENERGY BOOSTER
Key Benefits
Ginseng, particularly PANAX GINSENG and AMERICAN GINSENG, is a NATURAL STIMULANT that supports ENERGY PRODUCTION and ADRENAL HEALTH. It's especially useful for individuals facing BURNOUT or recovering from PROLONGED STRESS.

This herb is shown to:

- NORMALIZE CORTISOL SECRETION.
- BOOST IMMUNE FUNCTION weakened by CHRONIC STRESS.
- IMPROVE MENTAL ALERTNESS and FOCUS.

How It Works
Ginsenosides, the ACTIVE COMPOUNDS in ginseng, influence the HYPOTHALAMUS to MODULATE CORTISOL RELEASE. They also support MITOCHONDRIAL FUNCTION, enhancing CELLULAR ENERGY PRODUCTION.

Safe Usage
- DOSAGE: 200–400 MG daily of a STANDARDIZED EXTRACT.
- TIMING: Morning consumption is ideal for ENERGY SUPPORT.
- PRECAUTIONS: Avoid use with BLOOD THINNERS or during HYPERTENSION, as it may INCREASE BLOOD PRESSURE.

HOLY BASIL: THE STRESS RELIEVER
Key Benefits
Known as TULSI in Ayurvedic traditions, HOLY BASIL is a MILD ADAPTOGEN that calms NERVOUS TENSION and promotes MENTAL CLARITY. It also offers ANTI-INFLAMMATORY and IMMUNE-BOOSTING effects.

Holy basil is effective for:
- LOWERING CORTISOL LEVELS during EMOTIONAL DISTRESS.
- EASING ANXIETY without causing DROWSINESS.
- SUPPORTING DIGESTIVE HEALTH, often disrupted by STRESS.

How It Works
Holy basil's URSOLIC ACID and ROSMARINIC ACID protect cells from OXIDATIVE DAMAGE while balancing NEUROTRANSMITTERS. It also helps regulate BLOOD SUGAR, preventing SPIKES that exacerbate STRESS.

Safe Usage
- DOSAGE: 300–500 MG per day or TEA INFUSIONS made with DRIED LEAVES.
- TIMING: Mid-morning or early evening.
- PRECAUTIONS: May lower BLOOD SUGAR levels—monitor if using DIABETES MEDICATIONS.

HOW TO USE HERBS SAFELY AND EFFECTIVELY

Start Slowly
Introduce ONE HERB at a time to MONITOR YOUR BODY'S RESPONSE. Adjust DOSAGES gradually and observe for POSITIVE EFFECTS or any SENSITIVITIES.

Rotate Adaptogens
Avoid LONG-TERM USE of a single adaptogen. Rotating herbs every 6–8 WEEKS prevents the body from DEVELOPING TOLERANCE and maintains EFFECTIVENESS.

Combine Wisely
Some adaptogens work best in COMBINATIONS. For example:
- ASHWAGANDHA and RHODIOLA balance ENERGY and CALMNESS.
- GINSENG and HOLY BASIL enhance MENTAL CLARITY and EMOTIONAL STABILITY.

Check Interactions
Always consult a HEALTH PROFESSIONAL before starting HERBAL SUPPLEMENTS, especially if taking MEDICATIONS or managing CHRONIC CONDITIONS.

Herbs and adaptogens are more than QUICK FIXES. They represent a LONG-TERM APPROACH to NURTURING RESILIENCE and BALANCE. When used MINDFULLY, these natural allies empower the body to handle LIFE'S STRESSORS while maintaining ENERGY and CLARITY.

7.2 SUPPLEMENTS AND ESSENTIAL OILS

The human body has an extraordinary capacity to handle STRESS, but prolonged exposure to physical, emotional, or environmental pressures can lead to CORTISOL IMBALANCES and leave the system OVERWORKED. Supplements and essential oils offer NATURAL TOOLS to NOURISH THE BODY, RESTORE EQUILIBRIUM, and CALM THE MIND. By targeting NUTRITIONAL DEFICIENCIES and activating the PARASYMPATHETIC NERVOUS SYSTEM, these approaches work holistically to SUPPORT STRESS REDUCTION.

Supplements such as MAGNESIUM, OMEGA-3 FATTY ACIDS, and VITAMIN C replenish DEPLETED NUTRIENTS and stabilize BIOCHEMICAL PROCESSES. Meanwhile, essential oils like LAVENDER, BERGAMOT, and CHAMOMILE interact directly with the OLFACTORY SYSTEM, influencing BRAIN CHEMISTRY and EMOTIONAL STATES. Together, these methods create a foundation for RESILIENCE and RECOVERY.

MAGNESIUM: THE RELAXATION MINERAL

Key Benefits
Magnesium is often referred to as the ANTI-STRESS MINERAL due to its ability to CALM THE NERVOUS SYSTEM, REDUCE MUSCLE TENSION, and ENHANCE SLEEP QUALITY. It plays a central role in over 300 ENZYMATIC PROCESSES that regulate ENERGY PRODUCTION, NERVE FUNCTION, and HORMONAL BALANCE.

When magnesium levels are LOW, the body becomes more REACTIVE TO STRESS, leading to TIGHT MUSCLES, IRRITABILITY, and INSOMNIA. Restoring magnesium levels can:

- LOWER CORTISOL LEVELS and improve HPA AXIS REGULATION.
- SUPPORT NEUROTRANSMITTERS like GABA that promote RELAXATION.
- REDUCE INFLAMMATION, which contributes to CHRONIC STRESS.

Sources and Forms
Magnesium comes in several forms, each with UNIQUE ABSORPTION RATES:

- MAGNESIUM GLYCINATE: Best for CALMNESS and SLEEP SUPPORT.
- MAGNESIUM CITRATE: Suitable for those who need DIGESTIVE SUPPORT.
- MAGNESIUM MALATE: Ideal for MUSCLE RELAXATION and ENERGY PRODUCTION.

Usage Guidelines
- DOSAGE: Most adults benefit from 300–400 MG per day.
- TIMING: Taken in the EVENING can enhance SLEEP QUALITY.
- PRECAUTIONS: Excessive doses may cause DIGESTIVE UPSET.

OMEGA-3 FATTY ACIDS: BRAIN AND MOOD STABILIZERS

Key Benefits
Omega-3 fatty acids, particularly EPA and DHA found in FISH OIL, are essential for BRAIN HEALTH and HORMONAL REGULATION. They reduce INFLAMMATION and support CELL MEMBRANE INTEGRITY, making them vital for NERVOUS SYSTEM STABILITY.

Research has linked omega-3s to:

- REDUCED CORTISOL SPIKES during STRESSFUL SITUATIONS.
- IMPROVED MOOD REGULATION and DECREASED SYMPTOMS of ANXIETY.
- ENHANCED FOCUS and COGNITIVE PERFORMANCE.

Sources and Forms
Natural sources include FATTY FISH like SALMON, MACKEREL, and SARDINES. Supplements can provide concentrated doses, available as:

- FISH OIL CAPSULES: High in EPA and DHA.
- ALGAE-BASED SUPPLEMENTS: A VEGAN ALTERNATIVE.
- FLAXSEED OIL: Rich in ALA, a precursor to EPA/DHA.

Usage Guidelines
- DOSAGE: 1000–3000 MG daily.
- TIMING: Take with MEALS to improve ABSORPTION.
- PRECAUTIONS: May interact with BLOOD THINNERS.

VITAMIN C: THE STRESS SHIELD

Key Benefits
Vitamin C is a POTENT ANTIOXIDANT that NEUTRALIZES FREE RADICALS produced during STRESS RESPONSES. It also supports ADRENAL FUNCTION, which is vital for CORTISOL REGULATION.

This vitamin has been shown to:

- LOWER CORTISOL LEVELS after ACUTE STRESS.
- ENHANCE IMMUNE FUNCTION, which can be weakened by CHRONIC STRESS.
- REDUCE FATIGUE and promote RECOVERY.

Sources and Forms
While fresh fruits like ORANGES, KIWIS, and STRAWBERRIES provide natural sources, supplementation can deliver HIGHER DOSES when needed.

Usage Guidelines
- DOSAGE: 500–2000 MG per day.
- TIMING: Splitting doses throughout the day improves ABSORPTION.
- PRECAUTIONS: Excessive doses may cause DIGESTIVE UPSET.

ESSENTIAL OILS: AROMATIC STRESS RELIEVERS
LAVENDER: THE ULTIMATE RELAXER
Lavender oil is RENOWNED for its ability to REDUCE ANXIETY, LOWER HEART RATES, and INDUCE CALMNESS. It interacts with GABA RECEPTORS in the brain, providing a MILD SEDATIVE EFFECT.

How to Use
- DIFFUSERS: Add 5–10 DROPS for AROMATIC INHALATION.
- TOPICAL APPLICATION: Mix with a CARRIER OIL and apply to PULSE POINTS.
- BATHS: Combine with EPSOM SALTS for a STRESS-RELIEVING SOAK.

BERGAMOT: THE UPLIFTING OIL
Bergamot has a CITRUS AROMA that promotes POSITIVITY and EMOTIONAL BALANCE. Studies have linked it to LOWERED CORTISOL and IMPROVED MOOD.

How to Use
- INHALATION: Add a few drops to TISSUE or a DIFFUSER.
- MASSAGE: Blend with JOJOBA OIL for a CALMING RUB.

CHAMOMILE: THE GENTLE SOOTHER
Chamomile offers ANTI-INFLAMMATORY and SEDATIVE EFFECTS. It's perfect for those experiencing RESTLESSNESS or MUSCLE TENSION.

How to Use
- TEA: Drink before BEDTIME.
- COMPRESSES: Apply to FOREHEAD or NECK to EASE TENSION.

COMBINING SUPPLEMENTS AND ESSENTIAL OILS FOR SYNERGY
BLENDING SUPPLEMENTS with AROMATHERAPY creates a MULTI-LAYERED APPROACH to stress relief. For example, pairing MAGNESIUM SUPPLEMENTATION with a LAVENDER-INFUSED BATH amplifies RELAXATION. Likewise, OMEGA-3S combined with BERGAMOT AROMATHERAPY can enhance MOOD STABILITY throughout the day.

PRACTICAL TIPS FOR DAILY USE
- CONSISTENCY MATTERS: Supplements and essential oils yield the best results when used REGULARLY.
- TRACK PROGRESS: Maintain a JOURNAL to monitor SYMPTOMS and ADJUST DOSAGES.
- LAYER STRATEGIES: Incorporate DIET, EXERCISE, and BREATHING TECHNIQUES alongside NATURAL REMEDIES.

By integrating TARGETED NUTRITION and AROMATHERAPY PRACTICES into daily routines, the BODY AND MIND become MORE RESILIENT, creating a sustainable foundation for LONG-TERM STRESS RELIEF.

7.3 DIY REMEDIES

When stress feels overwhelming, simple DO-IT-YOURSELF (DIY) REMEDIES can offer a sense of CONTROL, COMFORT, and RELIEF. Crafting your own stress-relief tools transforms ordinary self-care into INTENTIONAL RITUALS that NURTURE BOTH BODY AND MIND. From AROMATIC SCRUBS and LUXURIOUS BATHS to HERBAL TEAS and SOOTHING BLENDS, these homemade solutions allow you to TAILOR TREATMENTS to your specific needs and preferences.

Whether you crave a REVITALIZING SCRUB to INVIGORATE TIRED SKIN or a STEAMING MUG OF HERBAL TEA to MELT TENSION, these recipes invite you to PAUSE, UNWIND, and RECONNECT with your inner calm.

STRESS-RELIEF SCRUBS: EXFOLIATION MEETS RELAXATION

Exfoliating scrubs not only REVITALIZE THE SKIN but also provide a SENSORY EXPERIENCE that helps DISTRACT THE MIND from worries. The combination of GENTLE TEXTURES, NATURAL OILS, and AROMATIC ESSENTIAL OILS creates a MULTISENSORY ESCAPE.

SOOTHING LAVENDER SUGAR SCRUB

INGREDIENTS:

- 1 cup GRANULATED SUGAR (for gentle exfoliation)
- ½ cup COCONUT OIL (for hydration)
- 10 drops LAVENDER ESSENTIAL OIL (for relaxation)
- 1 tablespoon DRIED LAVENDER BUDS (optional, for texture)

INSTRUCTIONS:

1. Combine the SUGAR and COCONUT OIL in a bowl until fully blended.
2. Add LAVENDER ESSENTIAL OIL and stir.
3. Mix in DRIED LAVENDER BUDS for added texture and fragrance.
4. Store in a GLASS JAR and use during showers to massage away STRESS AND TENSION.

Benefits:

- Lavender's CALMING SCENT lowers CORTISOL LEVELS and promotes SERENITY.
- Coconut oil leaves skin HYDRATED and NOURISHED.
- Gentle exfoliation boosts CIRCULATION, easing MUSCLE STIFFNESS.

INVIGORATING CITRUS COFFEE SCRUB

INGREDIENTS:

- ½ cup GROUND COFFEE (for exfoliation and circulation)
- ½ cup BROWN SUGAR (softens rough skin)
- 1/3 cup ALMOND OIL (moisturizes deeply)
- 8 drops ORANGE ESSENTIAL OIL (uplifts mood)

INSTRUCTIONS:

1. Mix COFFEE GROUNDS and BROWN SUGAR in a bowl.
2. Add ALMOND OIL and stir to create a paste.
3. Incorporate ORANGE ESSENTIAL OIL for a BRIGHTENING AROMA.
4. Massage into DAMP SKIN during showers, focusing on TENSE AREAS.

Benefits:

- Coffee's natural CAFFEINE CONTENT reduces INFLAMMATION and BOOSTS CIRCULATION.
- Orange oil energizes while providing STRESS-RELIEVING PROPERTIES.
- The scrub leaves skin SMOOTH and REVITALIZED.

BATH RITUALS: IMMERSIVE RELAXATION THERAPY

A warm bath can lower cortisol levels, ease muscle tension, and promote sleep. Adding essential oils, herbs, and mineral SALTS transforms bath time into a HEALING PRACTICE.

ROSE AND CHAMOMILE MILK BATH

INGREDIENTS:

- 1 cup POWDERED MILK (soothes and softens skin)
- ½ cup EPSOM SALT (relaxes muscles)
- 10 drops CHAMOMILE ESSENTIAL OIL (calms nerves)
- 5 drops ROSE ESSENTIAL OIL (elevates mood)
- ¼ cup DRIED ROSE PETALS (optional, for elegance)

INSTRUCTIONS:

1. Combine all dry ingredients in a bowl.
2. Add ESSENTIAL OILS and stir well.
3. Pour the mixture into WARM BATHWATER.
4. Soak for 20–30 MINUTES, inhaling the AROMATIC VAPORS.

Benefits:

- Chamomile reduces ANXIETY and promotes RELAXATION.
- Epsom salts replenish MAGNESIUM LEVELS, easing MUSCLE TENSION.
- Rose essential oil provides an UPLIFTING AROMA that supports EMOTIONAL BALANCE.

HERBAL TEAS: SIPPING CALMNESS

Herbal teas act as GENTLE REMEDIES to SOOTHE THE NERVOUS SYSTEM. Drinking warm infusions creates a RITUAL OF SLOWING DOWN and RECONNECTING with the present moment.

CHAMOMILE AND LEMON BALM TEA

INGREDIENTS:

- 1 teaspoon DRIED CHAMOMILE FLOWERS
- 1 teaspoon DRIED LEMON BALM LEAVES
- 1 teaspoon RAW HONEY (optional, for sweetness)
- 1 cup BOILING WATER

INSTRUCTIONS:

1. Add CHAMOMILE and LEMON BALM to a TEA INFUSER or TEAPOT.
2. Pour BOILING WATER over the herbs and let steep for 5–7 MINUTES.
3. Strain and add HONEY if desired.
4. Sip slowly, allowing the AROMA and FLAVOR to ease TENSION.

Benefits:

- Chamomile reduces NERVOUS TENSION and encourages RESTFUL SLEEP.
- Lemon balm acts as a NATURAL SEDATIVE and MOOD ENHANCER.

AROMATHERAPY BLENDS: PORTABLE CALM

Aromatherapy blends offer on-the-go stress relief that fits into busy lifestyles. Small roller bottles and sprays can be used throughout the day to RESET EMOTIONS.

CALM AND FOCUS ROLL-ON BLEND

INGREDIENTS:
- 10 ml JOJOBA OIL (carrier oil)
- 5 drops FRANKINCENSE ESSENTIAL OIL (centers the mind)
- 5 drops BERGAMOT ESSENTIAL OIL (uplifts mood)
- 3 drops PEPPERMINT ESSENTIAL OIL (energizes without overstimulation)

INSTRUCTIONS:
1. Combine oils in a ROLLER BOTTLE.
2. Shake gently to blend.
3. Apply to WRISTS, NECK, or TEMPLES as needed.

Benefits:
- Frankincense supports MENTAL CLARITY.
- Bergamot provides EMOTIONAL BALANCE.
- Peppermint refreshes and STIMULATES FOCUS.

PERSONALIZING YOUR DIY REMEDIES

Crafting stress-relief remedies invites you to EXPERIMENT and DISCOVER WHAT RESONATES MOST. Customize ingredients to match your MOOD, SEASON, or SPECIFIC NEEDS. Whether you seek CALM BEFORE BED or a MIDDAY BOOST, these DIY options can EMPOWER YOU to take charge of your WELL-BEING.

From scrubs that AWAKEN THE SENSES to teas that NURTURE THE SOUL, each remedy becomes a DAILY RITUAL for cultivating PEACE AND BALANCE.

Conclusion to Chapter 7: Natural Support for Stress Reduction

The journey to STRESS RELIEF doesn't have to be complicated or overwhelming. By integrating HERBAL REMEDIES, NUTRITIONAL SUPPLEMENTS, and AROMATHERAPY BLENDS into your self-care routine, you can access POWERFUL TOOLS that CALM THE NERVOUS SYSTEM, REDUCE CORTISOL LEVELS, and NURTURE EMOTIONAL BALANCE.

The strategies explored in this chapter are designed to fit SEAMLESSLY into daily life—whether through a QUICK MINDFULNESS TEA, a SOOTHING BATH, or an INVIGORATING SCRUB. Small, CONSISTENT ACTIONS can create LASTING CHANGES, offering not just relief but also RENEWED ENERGY and CLARITY.

As you explore these remedies, remember that PERSONALIZATION IS KEY. Pay attention to how your body responds and ADJUST YOUR APPROACH as needed. Nature's solutions are GENTLE YET EFFECTIVE, giving you the freedom to create a TOOLBOX OF SUPPORT that evolves with your needs—helping you RECLAIM CALMNESS and BUILD RESILIENCE one step at a time.

CHAPTER 8: LONG-TERM STRATEGIES FOR A LOW-STRESS LIFE

In today's fast-paced world, stress has become more than just an occasional challenge—it's a constant presence, quietly influencing how we think, feel, and function. While quick fixes may offer temporary relief, achieving *lasting calm* requires more than short-term solutions. It demands a shift in how we approach our lives, from the foods we eat to the habits we nurture and the environments we create.

This chapter explores *proven strategies* to help you maintain balanced cortisol levels and build resilience against future stressors. These aren't rigid systems or one-size-fits-all formulas. Instead, they're *flexible frameworks* designed to integrate seamlessly into your lifestyle—whether you're a busy parent, a high-performing professional, or someone simply seeking a sense of control.

You'll learn how to craft daily rituals that naturally lower stress, strengthen your body's defenses, and promote emotional stability. From designing calming spaces to fostering supportive relationships and practicing mindful living, the focus is on creating *sustainable habits* that protect your well-being over time.

True transformation doesn't happen overnight, but with the *right tools and mindset*, you can reclaim balance, restore vitality, and live a life that feels as good as it looks.

8.1 DESIGNING AN ANTI-STRESS LIFESTYLE

Creating a LOW-STRESS LIFESTYLE isn't about eliminating challenges or living in isolation. Instead, it's about DESIGNING DAILY HABITS and INTENTIONAL CHOICES that build RESILIENCE, BALANCE CORTISOL LEVELS, and ENHANCE EMOTIONAL STABILITY. This process requires a PROACTIVE MINDSET—one that emphasizes PREVENTION rather than REACTION. By identifying COMMON TRIGGERS, incorporating REGENERATIVE BREAKS, and prioritizing RECOVERY, it becomes possible to build a SUSTAINABLE FOUNDATION for long-term well-being.

This section explores how to RESTRUCTURE ROUTINES, ADJUST PRIORITIES, and FINE-TUNE BEHAVIORS to create an environment that supports MENTAL CLARITY and PHYSICAL RELAXATION. It also highlights PRACTICAL METHODS to protect your ENERGY RESERVES and EMOTIONAL HEALTH through MINDFUL STRATEGIES that address modern stressors.

RECOGNIZING AND AVOIDING HIDDEN STRESS TRIGGERS

Stress often arises not from SINGLE DRAMATIC EVENTS but from SUBTLE, RECURRING PRESSURES that accumulate over time. These HIDDEN STRESSORS may include OVERCOMMITMENT, POOR TIME MANAGEMENT, DIGITAL OVERLOAD, and ENVIRONMENTAL CLUTTER. While these factors might seem HARMLESS at first, their CUMULATIVE EFFECT can spike CORTISOL LEVELS and leave the body in a CONSTANT STATE OF ALERT.

DIGITAL NOISE AND INFORMATION OVERLOAD

Today's world is dominated by CONSTANT NOTIFICATIONS, EMAILS, and SOCIAL MEDIA FEEDS. This DIGITAL NOISE bombards the brain with STIMULI, making it difficult to UNPLUG and UNWIND. The key to managing DIGITAL OVERLOAD is to SET BOUNDARIES.

- SCHEDULE SCREEN-FREE TIMES during meals, mornings, and evenings.
- Use FOCUS APPS to block distractions when working.
- Establish DESIGNATED ZONES at home that are TECH-FREE.

OVERCOMMITTING AND SAYING YES TOO OFTEN

Modern lifestyles often glorify BUSYNESS, leading to OVERCOMMITMENT and MENTAL EXHAUSTION. People frequently say "yes" to requests out of OBLIGATION, only to feel RESENTFUL and BURNED OUT. Learning to say NO without guilt can protect MENTAL BANDWIDTH and allow for INTENTIONAL REST.

- Use phrases like "LET ME CHECK MY SCHEDULE FIRST" before agreeing to plans.
- Prioritize QUALITY OVER QUANTITY—focus on meaningful commitments.
- Block out PERSONAL RECHARGE TIME in your calendar as NON-NEGOTIABLE.

PHYSICAL CLUTTER AND ENVIRONMENTAL STRESS
Cluttered spaces can create VISUAL CHAOS and make it harder to RELAX. Studies show that DISORGANIZED ENVIRONMENTS lead to HIGHER CORTISOL LEVELS and REDUCED FOCUS. A simple way to minimize ENVIRONMENTAL STRESS is by DECLUTTERING AND ORGANIZING.

- Start small—clear one drawer or surface at a time.
- Invest in STORAGE SOLUTIONS to create an ORGANIZED ATMOSPHERE.
- Add PLANTS, SOFT LIGHTING, and NATURAL TEXTURES to make your home a CALMING RETREAT.

THE POWER OF SCHEDULED REST AND REGENERATIVE BREAKS
In the pursuit of productivity, people often overlook the importance of rest. Yet, the body's natural rhythms depend on periods of recovery to reset cortisol levels and recharge energy reserves. Implementing intentional breaks throughout the day allows both the MIND and BODY to stay BALANCED.

MICRO-BREAKS TO RESET THE NERVOUS SYSTEM
Instead of waiting until BURNOUT strikes, incorporating MICRO-BREAKS into daily routines helps prevent FATIGUE and improves FOCUS. These short pauses give the NERVOUS SYSTEM a chance to RECOVER and RESET.

- Take a 5-MINUTE WALK outdoors to RECONNECT WITH NATURE.
- Practice DEEP BREATHING EXERCISES to LOWER HEART RATE and EASE TENSION.
- Use the 20-20-20 RULE—every 20 minutes, look at something 20 feet away for 20 seconds.

WEEKLY REST DAYS FOR EMOTIONAL DETOX
Scheduling one day each week for INTENTIONAL REST promotes PHYSICAL RECOVERY and MENTAL CLARITY. Known as "RECOVERY DAYS," these periods offer space to STEP BACK from obligations and RECHARGE.

- Dedicate Sundays or a chosen day as a TECHNOLOGY-FREE ZONE.
- Engage in SLOW, NOURISHING ACTIVITIES like YOGA, JOURNALING, or CREATIVE HOBBIES.
- Treat these days as APPOINTMENTS WITH YOURSELF—non-negotiable time for SELF-CARE.

SEASONAL RETREATS FOR DEEP RESTORATION
Periodic GETAWAYS or RETREATS allow for DEEPER REJUVENATION. These breaks provide an opportunity to DISCONNECT from daily stressors and focus entirely on HEALING PRACTICES.

- Plan NATURE RETREATS to immerse yourself in CALMING ENVIRONMENTS.
- Attend WELLNESS WORKSHOPS or MEDITATION RETREATS to build NEW SKILLS.
- Use these trips as a way to REFLECT and REALIGN PRIORITIES.

CREATING A HOLISTIC STRESS-MANAGEMENT FRAMEWORK
Sustainable stress management goes beyond isolated habits. It's about weaving healthy rituals into every aspect of life—from how you wake up to how you unwind. This framework integrates mindful practices, nutritional support, and INTENTIONAL BOUNDARIES to create LONG-LASTING BALANCE.

MORNING ANCHORS FOR A CALM START
Starting the day with CLARITY can influence the ENTIRE MOOD. Create MORNING RITUALS that foster PEACE and FOCUS.

- Begin with STRETCHING or BREATHWORK to RELEASE TENSION.
- Follow with a NUTRIENT-RICH BREAKFAST to STABILIZE BLOOD SUGAR.
- Use AFFIRMATIONS to set a POSITIVE TONE for the day.

EVENING WIND-DOWN RITUALS

Just as mornings shape the day, EVENING ROUTINES determine SLEEP QUALITY and OVERNIGHT CORTISOL REGULATION.

- Dim lights an hour before bed to CUE RELAXATION.
- Take a WARM BATH with ESSENTIAL OILS to SOOTHE MUSCLES.
- Unplug from devices and read a CALMING BOOK.

THE ROLE OF CONSISTENCY IN STRESS RESILIENCE

Long-term stress reduction depends on CONSISTENCY. While it's tempting to seek QUICK FIXES, the most effective results come from HABITUAL PRACTICES. Building a LOW-STRESS LIFESTYLE means SHOWING UP DAILY for yourself, even when progress feels SLOW.

- Track patterns with a STRESS JOURNAL to notice TRIGGERS.
- Celebrate SMALL IMPROVEMENTS—better sleep, improved focus, or fewer mood swings.
- Adjust strategies based on LIFE CHANGES without guilt.

FINAL THOUGHTS ON DESIGNING AN ANTI-STRESS LIFESTYLE

Designing a LOW-STRESS LIFE is not about PERFECTION—it's about PROGRESS. By addressing HIDDEN TRIGGERS, embracing RESTORATIVE BREAKS, and building INTENTIONAL HABITS, it's possible to create STABILITY that lasts. Each practice, whether it's a FIVE-MINUTE MINDFULNESS BREAK or a WEEKLY RETREAT, forms part of a BIGGER PICTURE—one that promotes HEALTH, HAPPINESS, and RESILIENCE in the face of life's challenges.

8.2 THE ROLE OF HEALTHY RELATIONSHIPS AND COMMUNITY

In our fast-paced, digitally driven world, it's easy to overlook the profound impact that HEALTHY RELATIONSHIPS and a STRONG SENSE OF COMMUNITY have on our overall well-being. SOCIAL CONNECTIONS are not just a luxury or a nice-to-have; they are a FUNDAMENTAL COMPONENT of a LOW-STRESS LIFESTYLE. The science behind this is clear: HUMANS ARE WIRED FOR CONNECTION, and nurturing our relationships plays a pivotal role in BALANCING HORMONES, ENHANCING EMOTIONAL HEALTH, and REDUCING STRESS.

Having a SUPPORT NETWORK—whether friends, family, colleagues, or even community groups—helps buffer the effects of stress. Positive relationships provide a SENSE OF SAFETY, BELONGING, and VALIDATION, which can directly influence how we handle adversity and stress. But it's not just about the quantity of connections; it's the QUALITY that matters. Meaningful relationships contribute to EMOTIONAL RESILIENCE, provide a SPACE FOR EXPRESSION, and can even offer PRACTICAL SUPPORT during difficult times. They can be instrumental in LOWERING CORTISOL LEVELS and BOOSTING OXYTOCIN, the "feel-good" hormone that counteracts stress.

Building and maintaining POSITIVE RELATIONSHIPS and a CONNECTED COMMUNITY can transform your ability to COPE WITH STRESS and increase your OVERALL HAPPINESS.

THE BIOLOGICAL AND PSYCHOLOGICAL BENEFITS OF HEALTHY RELATIONSHIPS

Before we dive into practical ways to foster POSITIVE RELATIONSHIPS and a SUPPORTIVE COMMUNITY, it's important to understand why these connections are so essential. Our bodies and minds are intricately designed to thrive in SOCIAL ENVIRONMENTS, and research has shown that our HORMONAL HEALTH is deeply influenced by the relationships we form.

HORMONAL IMPACT: THE POWER OF OXYTOCIN AND CORTISOL REGULATION

The STRESS RESPONSE is triggered by the hormone CORTISOL, which is released when we encounter challenges. While cortisol is crucial for SHORT-TERM SURVIVAL, chronic high levels can wreak havoc on our health. Long-term stress, in fact, contributes to numerous health problems, including HEART DISEASE, DIGESTIVE ISSUES, SLEEP DISTURBANCES, and WEAKENED IMMUNITY.

However, having SUPPORTIVE RELATIONSHIPS can act as a counterbalance. Positive interactions with loved ones release OXYTOCIN, often called the "bonding hormone," which has the opposite effect of cortisol. Oxytocin not only helps to REDUCE STRESS but also ENHANCES FEELINGS OF TRUST, EMPATHY, and CONNECTION. This creates a virtuous cycle: THE MORE SUPPORTED WE FEEL, the lower our cortisol levels, and the MORE RESILIENT WE BECOME in the face of challenges.

Studies have shown that people with strong social connections tend to have LOWER LEVELS OF STRESS, experience fewer MENTAL HEALTH ISSUES, and are better equipped to handle adversity. A HEALTHY RELATIONSHIP doesn't just soothe the mind—it impacts the PHYSICAL BODY, fostering an environment where HEALING AND REGENERATION are more likely to occur.

PSYCHOLOGICAL HEALTH: EMOTIONAL VALIDATION AND SUPPORT

At the psychological level, relationships offer a vital source of EMOTIONAL REGULATION. Stress tends to trigger negative thoughts, leading to feelings of HELPLESSNESS, OVERWHELM, or ANXIETY. Having someone to talk to—a friend, partner, or therapist—provides a SAFE SPACE to process these emotions, reducing their intensity. The simple act of expressing your feelings can help you gain CLARITY and PERSPECTIVE, making it easier to cope with stressful situations.

In times of crisis or difficulty, people who feel EMOTIONALLY SUPPORTED are more likely to develop ADAPTIVE COPING MECHANISMS, rather than resorting to DESTRUCTIVE BEHAVIORS. The presence of a caring friend or family member provides EMOTIONAL VALIDATION, letting you know that your struggles are not only UNDERSTOOD but also SHARED. This kind of support fosters SELF-COMPASSION and reduces the feelings of isolation that often accompany stress.

BUILDING POSITIVE CONNECTIONS: THE ART OF NURTURING RELATIONSHIPS

Creating and maintaining healthy, supportive relationships takes INTENTIONAL EFFORT and MINDFUL PRACTICE. In today's world, we often find ourselves distracted by TECHNOLOGY or overwhelmed by the demands of WORK and DAILY LIFE. However, by being deliberate in our approach to socializing and investing time in the people who truly matter, we can build a SOLID NETWORK of relationships that will help sustain us during stressful times.

QUALITY OVER QUANTITY: MEANINGFUL CONNECTIONS VS. SURFACE-LEVEL INTERACTIONS

In the age of SOCIAL MEDIA, it's easy to confuse CONNECTIONS with RELATIONSHIPS. While having a large circle of online friends can make us feel connected, these interactions often lack the depth required to create true emotional support. Meaningful relationships are built on TRUST, VULNERABILITY, and SHARED EXPERIENCES. They are relationships that nourish the soul and provide genuine EMOTIONAL SUPPORT during both good and bad times.

To create these types of connections, focus on the QUALITY of your relationships rather than the QUANTITY. A few deeply fulfilling connections can be more beneficial for your MENTAL HEALTH than a large network of superficial acquaintances. Here are some ways to build strong, meaningful relationships:

- **Prioritize face-to-face interactions**: While digital communication is convenient, in-person connections often create deeper bonds. Try to SCHEDULE REGULAR MEETUPS or even VIRTUAL FACE-TO-FACE CHATS.
- **Practice active listening**: When engaging in conversations, give your full attention to the person speaking. Show empathy and understanding, which creates a sense of safety and support.
- **Be vulnerable**: Share your thoughts and feelings openly. Authenticity invites trust and fosters deeper emotional connections.

STRENGTHENING EXISTING RELATIONSHIPS
If you already have strong relationships in your life, it's essential to continue nurturing them. As time passes, even the closest bonds can become strained if not maintained. Regularly investing in existing relationships ensures that they remain supportive and resilient.

- **Check in regularly**: Make an effort to stay connected, even if it's just sending a text or making a quick call.
- **Celebrate milestones**: Whether it's a birthday, a promotion, or a personal achievement, celebrating the good moments strengthens bonds.
- **Offer support during tough times**: Sometimes, offering a listening ear or a helping hand during challenging periods deepens the connection between individuals.

THE ROLE OF COMMUNITY IN REDUCING STRESS
Beyond individual relationships, being part of a larger COMMUNITY provides an added layer of support that can be incredibly powerful in reducing stress. A strong community fosters a sense of BELONGING, PURPOSE, and SHARED GOALS. When we feel connected to a group, whether it's through a hobby, a faith group, or a social cause, it helps create a feeling of SAFETY and TRUST, which in turn lowers CORTISOL LEVELS.

FINDING THE RIGHT COMMUNITY FOR YOU
Building a supportive community involves finding spaces where you feel ACCEPTED and UNDERSTOOD. These communities might include:

- **Social groups**: Joining clubs or interest groups that share your passions can provide a sense of connection and allow you to unwind in a NON-JUDGMENTAL ENVIRONMENT.
- **Faith-based communities**: Many people find comfort and stability in religious or spiritual groups. These communities often provide emotional and practical support during difficult times.
- **Volunteering and giving back**: Helping others not only benefits those in need but also contributes to a SENSE OF PURPOSE and FULFILLMENT.

THE POWER OF COLLECTIVE HEALING
Communities also offer the opportunity for COLLECTIVE HEALING. The shared energy of a group can be incredibly RESTORATIVE and provide a sense of SHARED RESPONSIBILITY for the emotional and physical well-being of others.

Whether it's participating in a group meditation session, joining a SUPPORT GROUP for a specific issue, or simply engaging in social activities, being part of a community strengthens our emotional resilience, making us better equipped to handle stress.

NAVIGATING TOXIC RELATIONSHIPS
While healthy relationships are essential for reducing stress, toxic relationships can have the opposite effect. These relationships, which often involve manipulation, emotional abuse, or neglect, can dramatically increase stress and DYSREGULATE HORMONES.

RECOGNIZING TOXIC PATTERNS
It's important to be aware of toxic dynamics, including:

- **Constant negativity**: When interactions with someone consistently leave you feeling DRAINED, UNAPPRECIATED, or EXHAUSTED, it's a red flag.
- **Emotional manipulation**: If you feel CONTROLLED or MANIPULATED in a relationship, it's time to reassess the connection.
- **Lack of support**: Healthy relationships are about MUTUAL SUPPORT. If someone is consistently UNSUPPORTIVE, or even DISMISSING your emotions, it may be a sign that the relationship is unhealthy.

SETTING BOUNDARIES AND LETTING GO
Sometimes, the best way to preserve your well-being is to DISTANCE YOURSELF from toxic people. Setting FIRM BOUNDARIES can help protect your emotional health, and in extreme cases, ENDING RELATIONSHIPS that consistently harm you may be necessary for healing.

Nurturing HEALTHY RELATIONSHIPS and building a supportive COMMUNITY is integral to creating a LOW-STRESS LIFESTYLE. By intentionally fostering positive connections, we can create an environment where EMOTIONAL HEALTH flourishes, STRESS diminishes, and our ability to THRIVE increases.

8.3 CELEBRATING PROGRESS AND STAYING MOTIVATED

Living a LOW-STRESS LIFESTYLE isn't about reaching a specific finish line—it's about building habits that keep you balanced and resilient over time. Whether you've just started making changes or you're months into your journey, CELEBRATING PROGRESS and STAYING MOTIVATED is essential for maintaining momentum. Progress, no matter how small, deserves recognition because it reinforces your efforts, strengthens your commitment, and builds confidence in your ability to handle life's challenges.

True transformation is about embracing growth as a process, not a destination. The key is to MEASURE SUCCESS IN WAYS THAT RESONATE WITH YOUR VALUES and focus on SMALL WINS that reflect meaningful change. Sustaining motivation requires a balance of SELF-AWARENESS, ADAPTABILITY, and SELF-COMPASSION, all of which keep you moving forward—even when setbacks occur.

REDEFINING SUCCESS: BEYOND THE SCALE AND SURFACE-LEVEL GOALS

When people think of self-improvement, it's often tied to VISIBLE OUTCOMES—a smaller waistline, a lower number on the scale, or a more sculpted physique. While these benchmarks might serve as SHORT-TERM MOTIVATORS, they rarely provide lasting satisfaction. Focusing solely on EXTERNAL ACHIEVEMENTS can make it easy to overlook the DEEPER CHANGES happening beneath the surface—the MENTAL CLARITY, EMOTIONAL RESILIENCE, and INNER PEACE you're cultivating.

SHIFTING TO INTERNAL SUCCESS MARKERS
Real success often shows up in ways that can't be measured by a mirror or a scale. It's the ability to RESPOND CALMLY to unexpected stress, the ENERGY you feel when you wake up, or the PEACE OF MIND that comes from feeling in control of your schedule. These internal changes may not be flashy, but they're powerful indicators that you're BUILDING A FOUNDATION for long-term well-being.

Ask yourself:

- Are you SLEEPING BETTER and waking up REFRESHED?
- Do you feel MORE FOCUSED and LESS OVERWHELMED during the day?
- Are you RECOVERING FASTER from stressful events?
- Have you developed HEALTHIER COPING MECHANISMS?

These are the victories worth celebrating because they reflect SUSTAINABLE PROGRESS. A calmer nervous system and improved hormonal balance often PRECEDE VISIBLE RESULTS. Recognizing and appreciating these shifts helps reinforce your habits and keep you MOTIVATED to continue.

TRACKING EMOTIONAL AND MENTAL GROWTH
Keeping a JOURNAL can be one of the most effective tools for measuring progress in areas that aren't easily quantified. Write down your MOOD PATTERNS, ENERGY LEVELS, and STRESS TRIGGERS. Over time, you'll start to notice patterns—perhaps you're LESS REACTIVE to conflict or QUICKER TO RECOVER after a challenging day. These insights are invaluable for RECOGNIZING GROWTH and identifying areas that need more attention.

THE POWER OF SMALL WINS: BUILDING MOMENTUM THROUGH TINY VICTORIES

Big changes don't happen overnight. They're the result of SMALL, CONSISTENT ACTIONS that build momentum. Celebrating these TINY VICTORIES helps RETRAIN YOUR BRAIN to associate growth with POSITIVE REINFORCEMENT, which keeps you motivated to continue.

THE PSYCHOLOGY BEHIND SMALL WINS

Research in BEHAVIORAL PSYCHOLOGY shows that CELEBRATING INCREMENTAL PROGRESS triggers the release of DOPAMINE, a neurotransmitter associated with PLEASURE and REWARD. This chemical boost reinforces the behavior, making it more likely to be repeated. Over time, this creates a FEEDBACK LOOP where small successes lead to bigger achievements.

For example:

- Replacing 15 MINUTES OF SOCIAL MEDIA SCROLLING with a MINDFUL BREATHING EXERCISE might seem minor, but it's a significant step toward REGAINING MENTAL CLARITY.
- Drinking a STRESS-RELIEF TEA before bed instead of relying on a glass of wine helps reinforce HEALTHIER COPING STRATEGIES.
- Saying NO to an unnecessary commitment strengthens your ability to SET BOUNDARIES and protect your time.

These actions build CONFIDENCE and signal to your brain that PROGRESS IS HAPPENING, even if it's not immediately visible.

MICRO-GOALS THAT KEEP YOU FOCUSED

Breaking larger goals into MANAGEABLE STEPS prevents overwhelm and makes success feel ATTAINABLE. Instead of aiming to "reduce stress completely," set a goal like:

- Practicing 5 MINUTES OF DEEP BREATHING every morning.
- Spending 10 MINUTES JOURNALING each night.
- Scheduling ONE SOCIAL ACTIVITY per week to foster connections.

Each time you complete one of these tasks, take a moment to ACKNOWLEDGE THE EFFORT. Over time, these actions become AUTOMATIC HABITS that support long-term well-being.

STAYING MOTIVATED DURING PLATEAUS AND SETBACKS

Even the most dedicated individuals face PLATEAUS—periods when progress slows or stalls. These moments can be discouraging, but they're a natural part of the GROWTH PROCESS. Staying motivated requires RESILIENCE and the ability to REFRAME CHALLENGES as opportunities for learning.

REFRAMING PLATEAUS AS GROWTH ZONES

Instead of viewing plateaus as failures, see them as CONSOLIDATION PHASES. Your body and mind may need time to ADJUST to the changes you've already made before moving forward. Use this time to REFLECT on what's working, CELEBRATE STABILITY, and FINE-TUNE YOUR APPROACH.

Ask yourself:

- What's improved since I started this journey?
- What's HOLDING ME BACK right now?
- What SMALL SHIFTS can I make to get back on track?

Often, SMALL TWEAKS—like adjusting your sleep schedule or adding a new mindfulness practice—can help REIGNITE PROGRESS.

BUILDING A REWARD SYSTEM THAT FUELS PROGRESS

Rewards are powerful tools for maintaining LONG-TERM MOTIVATION. However, it's important to choose rewards that ALIGN WITH YOUR GOALS and reinforce HEALTHY BEHAVIORS.

EXAMPLES OF HEALTHY REWARDS
- Treat yourself to a MASSAGE or SPA DAY after reaching a milestone.
- Invest in a NEW BOOK or COURSE that supports your growth.
- Plan a WEEKEND GETAWAY to recharge and celebrate your commitment to self-care.
- Buy a NEW JOURNAL or PLANNER to continue organizing your life intentionally.

These rewards remind you that SELF-CARE IS WORTH PRIORITIZING and encourage you to STAY FOCUSED on your path.

FINDING INSPIRATION THROUGH ROLE MODELS AND ACCOUNTABILITY

Staying motivated often requires looking outside yourself for INSPIRATION and ACCOUNTABILITY. Surround yourself with people who EMBODY THE MINDSET YOU WANT TO CULTIVATE and seek out communities that UPLIFT AND MOTIVATE YOU.

HOW TO STAY INSPIRED
- Follow podcasts, books, or speakers who focus on PERSONAL GROWTH and STRESS MANAGEMENT.
- Join ONLINE FORUMS or SUPPORT GROUPS where you can share successes and learn from others.
- Partner with an ACCOUNTABILITY BUDDY to set weekly goals and celebrate wins together.
- Having a SUPPORT SYSTEM keeps you grounded and reminds you that YOU'RE NOT ALONE in your journey.

Maintaining motivation isn't about pushing yourself relentlessly—it's about CELEBRATING PROGRESS, EMBRACING GROWTH, and STAYING FLEXIBLE. Every small win is proof that you're building a FOUNDATION FOR RESILIENCE—one choice at a time.

Conclusion to Chapter 8: Long-Term Strategies for a Low-Stress Life

Lasting stress relief isn't about perfection—it's about CONSISTENCY. The strategies in this chapter are designed to be practical, realistic, and adaptable, empowering you to make meaningful changes without feeling overwhelmed.

By incorporating MINDFUL HABITS, optimizing your environment, and nourishing your body with supportive foods and practices, you've laid the groundwork for LONG-TERM BALANCE. Small, intentional actions—when repeated—become POWERFUL HABITS that shape your well-being from the inside out.

Remember, stress management isn't a destination; it's a LIFELONG JOURNEY. Be patient with yourself as you experiment with these approaches, and give yourself permission to grow through setbacks. The more you prioritize CALM AND CLARITY, the more natural it will feel to stay grounded, no matter what life throws your way.

Now it's time to take these tools and start living with PURPOSE, PEACE, AND RESILIENCE.

CONCLUSIONS

MAINTAINING BALANCE AFTER THE DETOX

Creating a LOW-STRESS LIFESTYLE is not a one-time event—it's a process of ONGOING REFINEMENT and INTENTION. Detoxing your body, mind, and habits marks the beginning, but maintaining balance requires CONSCIOUS CHOICES and CONSISTENT EFFORT. As life inevitably shifts and throws unexpected challenges, the ability to ADAPT while staying grounded becomes your greatest strength.

Stress management isn't about ELIMINATING PRESSURE COMPLETELY. Instead, it's about BUILDING RESILIENCE so that stress no longer controls your emotions, decisions, or well-being. This journey is less about PERFECTION and more about FLEXIBILITY. Balance is not static—it's fluid, requiring you to PIVOT and RECENTER as needed.

SUSTAINING THE RITUALS THAT ANCHOR YOU

Daily rituals act as ANCHORS, keeping you steady even when life feels turbulent. Whether it's starting the morning with MINDFUL BREATHING, ending the day with GRATITUDE JOURNALING, or prioritizing MOVEMENT to release tension, rituals transform INTENTIONS INTO HABITS.

CHOOSING PRACTICES THAT ALIGN WITH YOUR VALUES

Sustainability begins with ALIGNMENT. When rituals reflect your CORE VALUES, they feel less like tasks and more like EXTENSIONS OF YOUR IDENTITY.

- If INNER PEACE is a priority, integrate activities like MEDITATION or NATURE WALKS.
- For those valuing CONNECTION, prioritize WEEKLY CHECK-INS with loved ones or group activities that foster COMMUNITY.
- If GROWTH drives you, commit to LEARNING—whether through books, podcasts, or courses that nurture curiosity.

The KEY TO SUSTAINABILITY isn't doing EVERYTHING PERFECTLY. It's about choosing A FEW RITUALS that resonate and giving yourself PERMISSION TO EVOLVE those practices as your needs shift.

RECOGNIZING STRESS BEFORE IT ESCALATES

Balance doesn't mean stress will disappear entirely. Instead, it equips you to SPOT THE WARNING SIGNS EARLY and respond PROACTIVELY. Stress often creeps in subtly—through IRRITABILITY, FATIGUE, or MENTAL FOG. Learning to LISTEN TO YOUR BODY and TRUST YOUR INSTINCTS helps you act before tension builds.

EARLY SIGNALS TO WATCH FOR

- Feeling OVERWHELMED by minor tasks.
- Difficulty CONCENTRATING or FORGETFULNESS.
- Disrupted SLEEP PATTERNS—either struggling to fall asleep or waking up frequently.
- Physical tension, especially in the JAW, SHOULDERS, or NECK.
- Increased cravings for SUGAR, CAFFEINE, or COMFORT FOODS.

By tuning into these cues, you can implement QUICK RESETS—a 10-MINUTE STRETCH, a BREATHING EXERCISE, or stepping outside for FRESH AIR. Treating stress in its EARLY STAGES prevents it from becoming CHRONIC and overwhelming.

How to Keep Growing Beyond the Detox

Growth doesn't stop when the detox ends. It continues as you REFINE HABITS, CHALLENGE YOURSELF, and EMBRACE NEW POSSIBILITIES. Progress is not linear—it's a series of STEPS FORWARD, PAUSES, and even TEMPORARY SETBACKS. What matters most is MOMENTUM.

ADOPTING A GROWTH MINDSET
Sustained growth hinges on PERSPECTIVE. People who thrive see challenges as OPPORTUNITIES rather than OBSTACLES. They treat MISTAKES as LEARNING EXPERIENCES and view CHANGE as an invitation to EVOLVE.

SHIFTING FOCUS FROM OUTCOMES TO EFFORT
Instead of obsessing over END RESULTS, focus on the PROCESS. Celebrate EFFORT, CONSISTENCY, and COURAGE—qualities that drive REAL TRANSFORMATION.

- Did you STICK TO YOUR BEDTIME ROUTINE even during a busy week?
- Did you SET BOUNDARIES in a difficult situation?
- Did you choose a HEALTHIER RESPONSE to stress?

These wins reflect GROWTH—even when results aren't IMMEDIATELY VISIBLE.

INVESTING IN PERSONAL DEVELOPMENT
Growth thrives in ENVIRONMENTS OF CURIOSITY. Committing to LIFELONG LEARNING keeps you ENGAGED and MOTIVATED. This might involve:

- Exploring BREATHWORK TECHNIQUES for deeper relaxation.
- Attending WORKSHOPS on stress reduction or emotional resilience.
- Reading books on NEUROSCIENCE to better understand your body's response to stress.
- Practicing JOURNALING PROMPTS that promote SELF-REFLECTION.

New knowledge keeps your TOOLKIT EXPANDING, making it easier to ADAPT as your needs evolve.

CELEBRATING MILESTONES TO REINFORCE GROWTH
Growth is more likely to stick when it's ACKNOWLEDGED. Take time to celebrate MILESTONES—big or small. Whether it's 30 DAYS of consistent morning meditations or OVERCOMING A CHALLENGING SITUATION with grace, every achievement deserves recognition.

CREATING RITUALS OF CELEBRATION
- Treat yourself to a SPA DAY or a NATURE RETREAT.
- Reflect on your journey in a GRATITUDE JOURNAL.
- Share your progress with someone who has SUPPORTED you.

Celebrating reinforces POSITIVE BEHAVIOR and strengthens your COMMITMENT to growth.

Staying Rooted During Transitions
Life doesn't pause, and transitions—whether CAREER CHANGES, RELATIONSHIP SHIFTS, or UNEXPECTED EVENTS—can test your balance. These periods require FLEXIBILITY without losing sight of your CORE VALUES.

RETURNING TO YOUR FOUNDATION
When routines unravel, return to the PRACTICES THAT CENTER YOU. Focus on SLEEP, NUTRITION, and MOVEMENT—the pillars that support resilience. Revisit your WHY—the reasons you chose this path—and let it GUIDE YOUR ACTIONS.

Final Thoughts: Building a Legacy of Calm
True change isn't just about FEELING BETTER TEMPORARILY. It's about building a LIFESTYLE that supports calm, confidence, and EMOTIONAL FREEDOM. The tools you've gathered aren't just strategies—they're INVESTMENTS in your well-being. They empower you to RESPOND THOUGHTFULLY rather than react impulsively, to PRIORITIZE YOURSELF without guilt, and to LIVE WITH INTENTION.

ACKNOWLEDGEMENTS

No journey is ever walked alone. Every insight shared in this book has been shaped by the experiences, stories, and WISDOM OF OTHERS. Gratitude extends to the RESEARCHERS, PRACTITIONERS, and EVERYDAY PEOPLE who've tested these approaches in their own lives and shared their lessons.

To you, the reader—thank you for trusting this process and COMMITTING TO YOURSELF. Your dedication to GROWTH and BALANCE is an inspiration, and your journey will undoubtedly inspire others.

Keep building habits that NOURISH YOU. Keep prioritizing PEACE and CONNECTION. And most importantly, keep believing in the power of SMALL STEPS to create BIG TRANSFORMATIONS.

Thank you for choosing this book as a resource on your wellness journey. To support you further, I'm excited to offer **exclusive bonuses** designed to help you reduce stress, optimize sleep, and restore balance:

Scan the QR Code Below to Access:
- ⇨ **DAILY AFFIRMATIONS FOR STRESS RELIEF (PDF)**
- ⇨ **THE ULTIMATE SLEEP OPTIMIZATION GUIDE (PDF)**
- ⇨ **CORTISOL DETOX CHEAT SHEETS (PDF)**
- ⇨ **MINDFULNESS & BREATHING TECHNIQUES WORKBOOK (PDF)**

Share Your Feedback!

If this book has made a positive impact on your life, I'd be truly grateful if you could share your thoughts.

Scan the QR Code Below to Leave a Review:
- ⇨ **HELP OTHERS DISCOVER THIS BOOK.**
- ⇨ **INSPIRE SOMEONE TO BEGIN THEIR OWN WELLNESS JOURNEY.**

Thank You!

It's an honor to be part of your journey toward **health**, **balance**, and **happiness**. Thank you for letting me share this experience with you.

Wishing you peace, energy, and endless possibilities!

Made in United States
Orlando, FL
04 May 2025